Fitness After 50

Walter H. Ettinger, MD

UMass Memorial Medical Center

Brenda S. Wright, PhD

INTERVENT USA

Steven N. Blair, PED

The Cooper Institute

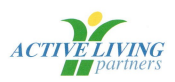
ACTIVE LIVING partners

HUMAN KINETICS

Library of Congress Cataloging-in-Publication Data

Ettinger, Walter H., 1951-
  Fitness after 50 / Walter H. Ettinger, Brenda S. Wright, Steven N. Blair.
      p. cm.
  Includes bibliographical references and index.
  ISBN 0-7360-4413-2 (soft cover)
  1. Middle-aged persons--Health and hygiene. 2. Physical fitness for middle-aged persons. 3. Exercise for middle-aged persons. I. Title: Fitness after fifty. II. Mitchell, Brenda S., 1946- III. Blair, Steven N. IV. Title.
  RA777.5.E878 2006
  613.7'0446--dc22

                            2005032105

ISBN-10: 0-7360-4413-2
ISBN-13: 978-0-7360-4413-4

Copyright © 2006 by Walter H. Ettinger, Brenda S. Wright, and Steven N. Blair

The Web addresses cited in this text were current as of December 2005, unless otherwise noted.

Acquisitions Editor: Michele Guerra, MS, CHES; **Developmental Editor:** Christine M. Drews; **Managing Editor:** Kathleen D. Bernard; **Copyeditor:** Bob Replinger; **Proofreader:** Kathy Bennett; **Indexer:** Sharon Duffy; **Permission Manager:** Carly Breeding; **Graphic Designer:** Nancy Rasmus; **Graphic Artist:** Yvonne Griffith; **Photo Manager:** Sarah Ritz; **Cover Designer:** Keith Blomberg; **Photographer (cover):** © Royalty Free / Corbis; **Photographer (interior):** Human Kinetics unless otherwise noted; **Art Manager:** Kelly Hendren; **Illustrator:** Keri Evans; **Printer:** Custom Color Graphics

Printed in the United States of America

10   9   8   7   6   5   4   3   2   1

Human Kinetics
Web site: www.HumanKinetics.com

United States: Human Kinetics
P.O. Box 5076
Champaign, IL 61825-5076
800-747-4457
e-mail: humank@hkusa.com

Canada: Human Kinetics
475 Devonshire Road Unit 100
Windsor, ON N8Y 2L5
800-465-7301 (in Canada only)
e-mail: orders@hkcanada.com

Europe: Human Kinetics
107 Bradford Road, Stanningley
Leeds LS28 6AT, United Kingdom
+44 (0) 113 255 5665
e-mail: hk@hkeurope.com

Australia: Human Kinetics
57A Price Avenue, Lower Mitcham
South Australia 5062
08 8277 1555
e-mail: liaw@hkaustralia.com

New Zealand: Human Kinetics
Division of Sports Distributors NZ Ltd.
P.O. Box 300 226 Albany
North Shore City
Auckland
0064 9 448 1207
e-mail: info@humankinetics.co.nz

Contents

Foreword   iv

Preface   v

Acknowledgments   ix

Introduction   xi

1   What's in It for You?   **1**

2   What You Think Matters   **21**

3   What's Age Got to Do With It?   **35**

4   Step It Up   **53**

5   Organize Yourself   **69**

6   Explore Aerobic Fitness   **89**

7   Find Places to Be Active   **113**

8   Get a Little Help From Your Friends   **129**

9   Create Your Aerobic Fitness Program   **139**

10   Add Strength, Balance, and Flexibility   **155**

11   Learn From Lapses and Manage Stress   **193**

12   Looking Ahead   **215**

Appendix   225

References   229

Word Search Solutions   231

Index   233

About the Authors   237

Foreword

It's been said that if exercise were a pill it would be the most widely used medicine in the Western world. We would willingly take this pill daily because of the enormous health benefits that this pill provides. We know that there is no pill, but we also know the reasons people would want it. At AARP we know that most people over 50 understand that exercise is good for them. They know it's the best thing they can do for their health. But what we've learned is that most people have a difficult time being active regularly. Lack of motivation, lack of time, worries about safety, and inclement weather are among the top barriers that are given. Oh, if only exercise were a pill.

Although there is nothing as simple as a pill, there is information that can help you do the real thing. *Fitness After 50* is a comprehensive guide that has something for everyone. Whether you are wanting to start a fitness program but don't know how to get going, or whether you have been trying for years to be active consistently but keep starting and stopping, or whether you have recently become more physically active and want to avoid the pitfalls from lapses, this book provides practical guidance.

The authors are experts who have spent years studying exercise behavior and have accumulated knowledge on what works and why as well as how the techniques can be applied. The authors are all over 50, so they bring personal insight on the changes and challenges that can influence our behavior and ability to exercise as we get older.

The book's friendly, nonjudgmental tone will encourage you to keep coming back. The exercises and sound advice in each chapter will help you find ways to get moving and keep moving. Follow the principles in this book and you'll reap the rewards of being fitter. You'll be dancing at your grandchildren's weddings, enjoying an independent life, and connecting with your community. So what are you waiting for? Isn't it time you began reading about the best medicine there is?

Margaret Hawkins, MS
Manager of Health Promotion
AARP

Preface

Welcome to *Fitness After 50!* We're glad that you chose this book. You are probably curious about becoming physically active, or perhaps you are already active and are looking for ways to bolster your physical activity plan. In any case, we have some exciting things to share with you. In *Fitness After 50,* we'll help you

- figure out how to get started,

- add variety and fun to your physical activities, and

- learn the skills that you'll need to keep on track when you run into trouble.

Fitness After 50 addresses the unique concerns that you may have as a middle-aged or older adult about your health and physical activity. Even if you are basically healthy, you may have to deal with conditions that are common after age 50—arthritis, osteoporosis, high blood pressure, or heart disease. As you look to start or change your physical activities, you may have some questions: Is it safe for me to increase my activity? What type of activity is best? How do I get started? How do I know whether I'm doing too much or not enough? If you're already active, you may want to know what you can do to add variety to your activity program. Or you may want to fine-tune your program to reap even more benefits.

You're sure to find answers to your questions in this book. Here are a few of the interesting and useful topics that we will address:

- Benefits and risks of physical activity for people over age 50, 70, and even 90

- How to be safe during activity

- How much physical activity is enough or too much

- Getting motivated to get moving

- Finding time for physical activity

- Deciding whether to do activity at home or at a fitness center

- Setting realistic goals
- Ways to be physically active without doing structured exercise
- Model programs for walking, water activities, stationary cycling, stretching, and strength building
- Developing an individualized plan
- Adapting physical activity programs for arthritis, osteoporosis, and other special conditions
- Knowing how and when to do more activity
- Activities to improve balance and prevent falls
- Using physical activity to relieve stress and improve mood
- Tracking progress
- Ways to get back on track if you lapse
- The role of physical activity in weight loss and weight control
- Sports, recreation, and leisure—new ways to be physically active
- How to be an advocate for physical activity in your community

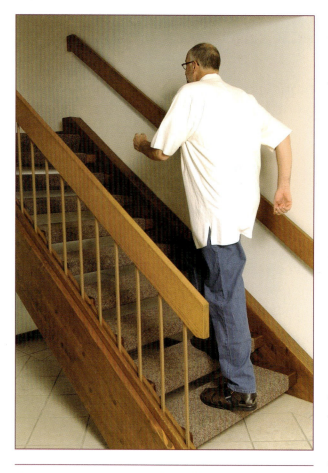

You can improve your health by making small changes, such as choosing to take the stairs!

A team of three—Dr. Walter Ettinger, Dr. Brenda Wright, and Dr. Steven Blair—wrote *Fitness After 50*. All of us were either approaching 50 or in our early 50s when our first collaborative book was published in 1996. We're older now, of course, and even more convinced of the merits of physical activity—for professional as well as personal reasons. Together we have 84 years of professional experience in the health and medical fields. We also have 116 years of combined participation in our own personal physical activity programs.

As you read the various chapters, you will likely recognize the voice of each of us. Walter is a medical doctor and university professor with a specialty in gerontology. He knows firsthand the real health issues for people over 50. He also sees the benefits that physical activity produces in the lives of his patients. Steve is a research scientist, an epidemiologist, who studies the relationships between physical activity and other lifestyle habits and health in large groups of people. He is the lead author of many frequently quoted research studies about the benefits of physical activity. He chaired the report on physical activity and health published by the U.S. surgeon general in 1996. Together, Steve and Walter provide the scientific and medical foundation that makes *Fitness After 50* a resource you can trust. Brenda is a health promotion consultant who has worked with corporations, hospitals and clinics, schools, government agencies, the military services, and resort and retirement communities to develop wellness programs. She has helped thousands of people adopt healthy lifestyles—to eat healthy, increase their physical activity, manage stress, stop smoking. You will recognize the influence of her background as a teacher as you read the book. Our reason for writing this book is simple: We want to be active and live independently for as long as possible. We want the same for our families, friends, and you, our readers. We believe in the old saying that physical activity "adds years to your life and life to your years."

Some of you who pick up this book will have tried to be physically active at some time in the past. If you've been disappointed in your previous attempts to get fit, this time can be different. We use an approach to physical activity that has been proved successful over and over with people just like you. It's never too late to get fit, and this book will help.

This book will work for you, whether you are just getting started or are already active. The chapters in this book are organized to help you increase your physical activity. Each chapter provides you with the structure, skills, and tools that you need to move along the path to greater motivation, more activity, and a higher level of fitness.

You will learn to use a variety of skills as you progress through this book. A skill that you learn in one chapter will be discussed again in a later chapter, but in a different way. You will apply previously used skills at future times. Building on what you have already learned and know will increase your likelihood of long-term success.

Fitness After 50 is designed as a self-paced workbook. Action boxes are a regular feature in every chapter. We will encourage you to answer

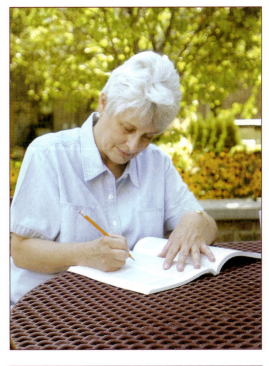

Work through *Fitness After 50* with pencil in hand. Feel free to write in your book.

questions, make lists, or complete logs as you read along. Keep a pen or pencil handy as you read and feel free to write in your book. Our experience tells us that people who get really involved with the tasks and tools in the book, especially if they are just getting started with physical activity, get more from the book and are more successful in staying active long term.

Other features bring the book to life. Personal profiles tell short stories about people over age 50, many just like you, at various activity and fitness levels, who are trying to increase their physical activity. Many have been successful in staying active. Others are still trying, learning from their experiences. Each chapter concludes with a chapter checklist—a list of ways to apply what you have learned to your everyday life. We've also included a word search puzzle in each chapter. See whether you can find words that highlight some of the key concepts in the chapters.

Thank you for purchasing *Fitness After 50*. We hope that you enjoy the book and the active lifestyle that it promotes.

Acknowledgments

We thank our colleagues at UMass Memorial Medical Center, INTER-VENT USA, and The Cooper Institute for their collaboration and stimulation over the years. The creative researchers for Project *Active* helped develop the lifestyle approach to physical activity that is featured prominently in this book. We are grateful for the leadership of a great group of interventionists involved in Project *Active,* especially Dr. Andrea Dunn, Dr. Bess Marcus, and Ruth Ann Carpenter.

Dr. James Prochaska, of the University of Rhode Island, and Dr. Carlo DiClemente, of the University of Maryland, Baltimore County, developed the stages of change model, the principal theoretical model supporting the strategies for increasing physical activity presented in this book. Dr. Bess Marcus, of Brown University, applied the stages of change model to the field of physical activity. Her recent book on motivational readiness, *Motivating People to Be Physically Active,* published by Human Kinetics, is a valuable resource. We acknowledge their contributions to our thinking.

Many medical, scientific, and public health organizations now recognize that the sedentary way of life that many people in industrialized countries follow, is an important health problem and are providing leadership in addressing this issue. We have enjoyed and continue to appreciate working with the American College of Sports Medicine; the American Heart Association; the American Alliance for Health, Physical Education, Recreation and Dance; the American Geriatrics Society; the National Coalition for the Promotion of Physical Activity; the Centers for Disease Control and Prevention; the National Institutes of Health; and the President's Council on Physical Fitness and Sports.

We are grateful to the National Institute on Aging and the National Heart, Lung, and Blood Institute for research support over the years. These grants have allowed us to develop our research program on the relation of physical activity and physical fitness to health and to explore new methods of helping sedentary people become more active.

We relied on the findings of surveys and interviews conducted by the AARP with people age 50 and over regarding their feelings, beliefs, needs, and interests related to exercise and physical activity. Following their example, we tried to give the book a voice that spoke to the reader in a positive, nonthreatening, nontechnical way.

For their contribution in shaping the content and thinking of this book, we thank a number of highly qualified reviewers: Julie McNeney, International Council on Active Aging (ICAA); Margaret Hawkins, MS, and staff at the AARP; Ruth Ann Carpenter, MS, RD, LD, The Cooper Institute; and Edward M. Phillips, MD, Harvard Department of Physical Medicine at Spaulding Rehabilitation Hospital.

A number of people contributed their time and expertise during the photo shoot for the book. We extend a special thanks to Sarah Ritz, photographer; Joyce Black, visual production assistant; and models Gaye Wong; Carolyn Casady-Trimble; and Gene Pitcher.

The combined efforts of a talented team at Human Kinetics gave the book physical reality. We appreciate that Rainer Martens, president of Human Kinetics, believes that *Fitness After 50* could complement the Active Living Partners programs. Special thanks go to Michele Guerra, director of Active Living Partners, and Christine Drews, senior developmental editor, who were involved in this project from its beginning. We are grateful for their patience in coordinating the efforts of three authors, which is never an easy task. In the end, we have a book that we can all be proud of and that we hope will be helpful to people over 50 who want to be more physically active.

Finally and most importantly, we thank our families who have provided love and support through the good times and the bad.

Introduction

Our approach to helping you become more active and fit is probably different from what you have tried in the past. Some health and fitness professionals promote programs that focus on immediate and dramatic results. Their approach assumes that when people decide they want to be more physically fit, they immediately take steps to be active. This action-oriented approach appeals to many people because they are looking for a quick fix. Thousands of people flock to programs that suggest they will look like bodybuilders after a few weeks of training. Many are quick to enroll in programs that promise significant weight loss in a few weeks. Although they should know better, people fall for these quick-fix programs. Unfortunately, most who attempt such programs are disappointed and ultimately give up on them. They ask, "Why didn't the program work? Where did I go wrong?"

How This Book Is Different

We will help you understand some basic principles about how people become and stay physically active. You'll begin by analyzing where you are along the path to regular physical activity. After considering your preferences and problems, you'll develop your personal plan. Then you'll put it into action. Using a try-and-try-again method, you will evaluate what works and what doesn't. If necessary, you will come up with a new plan and try again.

We believe that it is a mistake to view physical activity as an either–or event: either active or inactive, with nothing in between. In this book, you will learn to view physical activity as a fluid concept. People are creatures of habit. Changing your lifestyle routine will require thought, planning, and several tries before success becomes permanent. Only a few people can decide to become active and immediately act on their decisions. Most of us find that gradually reshaping habits and slowly building on success is a better and more realistic way to adopt a new habit. Everyone moves back and forth along the path between being very inactive and very active. Even people who have been active for years will at times not be as active as they might like. If you follow the step-by-step approach outlined in this book, you will progress to the point where you can maintain a moderately active lifestyle most, although probably not all, of the time.

Two Types of Physical Activity

Physical activity is all movement that uses energy. Using this definition, even fidgeting qualifies as physical activity. *Lifestyle physical activity* and *structured exercise* are two types of physical activity. Both can be effective in improving your health. Lifestyle activity includes taking the stairs, walking to do errands, and working in your yard—all the ways in which you are active in your everyday life. You can work lifestyle physical activity in throughout the day. You don't have to change clothes, go to a special place, or take a shower when you are done. No real costs are involved in lifestyle physical activity.

Structured exercise is repetitive physical activity done to improve physical fitness. Structured exercise includes group fitness classes, walking, swimming, cycling, jogging, lifting weights, stretching, yoga, and all active sports. People generally set aside a specific time of day to do structured exercise.

In *Fitness After 50,* you'll learn the skills you need to fit either type of physical activity into your daily life. You don't have to do structured exercise to become more active and fit.

Stages of Change

We believe that adopting an active lifestyle occurs in stages rather than all at once. Scientists who have studied the change process in thousands of people have observed that people change their habits gradually. They progress through a series of stages of change. Scientists have identified five stages of change. The major premise of the stages of change model is that people are at varying degrees of readiness to change at any time. Each stage in the process of change begins with a mind-set.

The five stages of change are described in table 1, along with a few of the feelings that people typically express in each stage. See whether you recognize yourself or others in these statements.

The names given to each stage of change make a lot of sense. People who are inactive and intend to stay that way are called precontemplators. Because contemplation means "thinking about," these people are not even

Table 1 Stages of Change

Stage	Statements by people in each stage
Precontemplation—Not even thinking about needing to be active or being resistant to starting to develop a plan for physical activity	"I'm fine. I don't need to be more active." "I'm too old to be active." "I've tried to be active in the past, but I couldn't stay with it. I'm not trying again."
Contemplation—Thinking about becoming more physically active now and then but not doing any activity	"I know I should be more active, but at my age, I'd feel foolish." "I don't know what to do to get started." "I'd like to be more active, but I'm afraid I might get injured."
Preparation—Developing a plan to become more active and being active from time to time, but not regularly	"I'm going to talk with my doctor about increasing my physical activity." "I've visited a health club that has special programs for people my age." "I'm enjoying taking short walks from time to time."
Action—Starting to be active on a regular basis but for less than six months	"I feel good when people notice that I'm more active." "Being active makes me feel better." "I hope I can stay active."
Maintenance—Staying regularly active for at least six months and feeling confident that you can stay physically active in the future	"I can't imagine not being physically active." "If I'm not able to be active, I really miss it." "I plan to be active for the rest of my life."

Prochaska and DiClemente first developed the stages of change model after studying people who stopped smoking, and Marcus further explored its application to physical activity (Prochaska and DiClemente 1983; Prochaska and Marcus 1994; Marcus and Forsyth 2003).

thinking about becoming more active. Some may not know that they need to be active, although it's difficult to imagine that people don't know that physical activity is good for them. Others may be resistant to starting to develop a habit of physical activity. The next stage, called contemplation, describes people who may be thinking about becoming active from time to time but are not ready to do anything. The third stage is called preparation. At this time, someone may be ready, willing, and planning to change, but not putting on walking shoes, at least not on most days. People in the next stage are ready and have taken action—they're off and walking (or cycling, swimming, or dancing) but still at risk for a setback. They haven't been active long enough to feel confident that they can stay with it for the long term. When people reach the point at which regular physical activity has become a habit and part of their personal value system, they are in the maintenance stage. They don't even think about not being active. They still have to negotiate obstacles—travel, family and job responsibilities, or a minor illness—that might interfere with their routine. People who pass into this last stage are likely to give up their inactive ways for good. They are committed to staying active for a lifetime.

You are probably wondering where you fit in these five stages. Chapter 1 begins with a short questionnaire to help you assess your current level of readiness to make a change toward a more active lifestyle. The answers that you give will indicate where you are in the five-stage process. Each stage of change is important, and all movement is progress. As you will learn, a lapse or setback can be an important learning opportunity that can help you build confidence to continue on the path to lifelong physical activity.

Skills for Change

To help you move from stage to stage, you'll use a variety of processes or skills. This book focuses more on skills than it does on stages. We believe that *skill power* is as important as *will power,* maybe even more important. We're not talking about physical skills, such as swinging a golf club or hitting a tennis ball. We're talking about skills related to what you know, think, and feel, as well as your actions (what you actually do).

People in different stages use different skills: People in early stages of change (contemplation and preparation) will rely more on the thinking and feeling skills. People in later stages (action and maintenance) will rely more on the doing and acting skills. This book has been designed to help people in all stages focus on the skills most important for them.

See the list of skills in table 2. These mental, emotional, and behavioral skills will be as important as any related to performing a specific activity or sport. Here's what we mean: You don't need to learn how to walk to start a walking program or go for a hike in the mountains. You already know how to walk! But you will need to learn how to select a good pair of walking shoes, find a safe and convenient place to walk, focus on making walking enjoyable, and then find time to be active every day or nearly day. You may need to know how to get help or support from others to put your plan in place. Or you may need to evaluate a situation and figure out how to adjust your plan. Learning lifestyle management skills will help you stay active long term.

A Self-Paced Program

You will move through this program at your own pace. Some people progress rapidly, whereas others take a long time to move from thinking about activity to making firm plans to starting an activity program. Knowing that you need to make a change and actually doing something to get started

Table 2 Skills for Becoming More Active

Thinking and feeling skills	Doing and acting skills
Becoming more knowledgeable—learning new information about physical activity	Changing your environment—making your surroundings supportive of your physical activity habits
Setting goals—setting realistic goals for physical activity	Monitoring your progress—keeping records of your physical activity; doing simple assessments to measure your improvement
Building confidence—believing that you can start and stay with a habit of regular physical activity	
Thinking differently—reviewing and challenging your thoughts and beliefs about physical activity	Managing time—finding time to be active regularly
	Managing stress—practicing stress management techniques
Recognizing cues—looking for things in yourself and your surroundings that promote or prevent physical activity	Building relationships—identifying and developing the support of others for your physical activity habits
Dealing with lapses—anticipating problems and planning ahead for times when it will be difficult to be active; thinking of ways to get back on track if you give up your activity for a time	Rewarding yourself—recognizing the progress that you make and celebrating successes for being active

are two different things. You can easily get stuck. A major objective of this book is to help you overcome the barriers that are keeping you from being more active.

If you are thinking about increasing your physical activity and are willing to make a serious attempt, you can move quickly to developing your plan. If you haven't been active in the recent past, you will need to spend some time figuring out what works best for you. Work thoughtfully through the first few chapters of this book. Rushing offers no advantage. You need time to develop your plan and arrange your surroundings to be supportive of physical activity. Even as you start to be active, you will need time to practice your new skills before they can become a habit. Be patient. Go at your own pace and give yourself ample time to lay a good foundation for the habits that you will practice for a lifetime. Becoming and staying physically active is a lifelong challenge.

Remember, changing your habits takes time and patience. You move forward and backward, and then go forward a little further. Lapses and setbacks are a natural and predictable part of the process and occur at every stage. Nearly everyone trying to be active has setbacks and lapses. Even people who have been active for quite a while get in a rut and become bored with their physical activity programs. For this reason, a spiral or

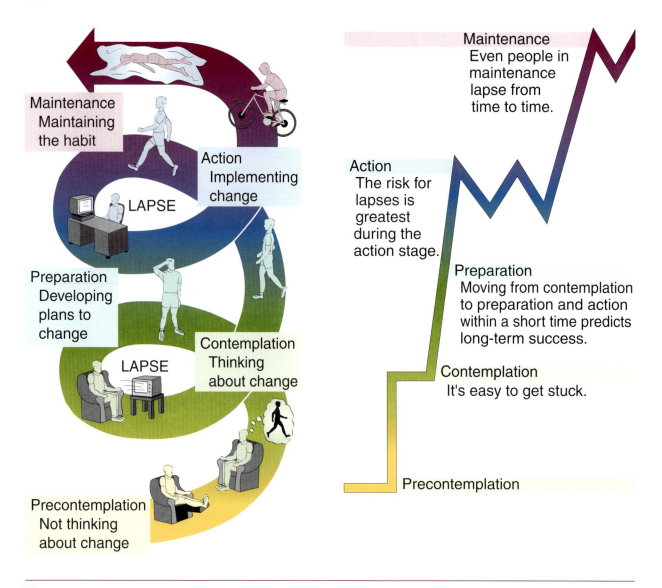

■ **Figure 1** When changing your habits, you will follow a path that looks like a spiral or a jagged line.

jagged line rather than a straight line is the best way to illustrate normal behavior change. Figure 1 shows the ideas. The process can be a bit like dancing the two-step—two steps forward and one step back.

Fortunately, most people who get off track don't go all the way back to square one. They learn from their experiences and, after some time, try new approaches and start making progress again. Managing lapses and preventing setbacks are critical aspects of adopting a new habit. This book will help you learn how to manage lapses and get quickly back on track to regular physical activity habits. You'll learn to figure out what tripped you up and what you can do differently next time to avoid a lapse. And you'll realize that you should give yourself credit for the progress that you've made. You are surely better off than when you started.

What Predicts Success

Because everyone is different, your path to physical activity will look different from that of anyone else. But several factors consistently predict success. Two—motivation and persistence—are key. You will learn much more about each of these and other factors in the chapters that follow, but here are a few points to think about now.

Lack of motivation is one of the top reasons people give for not being active. But where does motivation come from? How do you get motivated to be active? A common myth is that motivation comes from an external source—another person or event. In reality, you are the only one who can motivate yourself. We will help you find ways within yourself to get and stay motivated to be active.

You'll need to be persistent, to keep on keeping on! Many people believe that failure breeds failure. Do you believe that people who have repeatedly failed learn a pattern of behavior that they cannot break? It's true that if you keep repeating techniques that have failed in the past, you are not likely to be successful in the future. But if you use a new and different approach and try again, you can break the pattern of failure. One of the best predictors of success in the future is the number of serious attempts to change in the past. The person who tries again—each time trying a different approach—is more likely to succeed with the next attempt.

You will not see the word *failure* in future chapters of this book. We will focus on solving problems and learning from mistakes. You will learn to view lapses or setbacks as learning opportunities. Change is possible. Don't believe the old saying "You can't teach an old dog new tricks." It's never too late to get fit. We've seen many people in their 70s and 80s successfully start and stay with regular programs of physical activity. You can do it too!

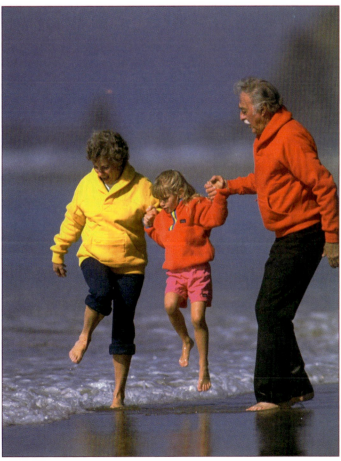

© Brian Drake/SportsChrome

You can be active and fit for a lifetime!

Summary

This book and our approach to helping you increase your physical activity are unique. Table 3 summarizes the differences between action-oriented and staged approaches to becoming physically active. Do you agree with us that the staged approach makes sense? Does this approach sound like one you would like to try?

We believe that our approach to physical activity offers a greater chance for long-term success than any other approach you may have tried. Thousands of people have used the strategies that you will use to become more active and change a variety of lifestyle habits.

So if you're thinking seriously about starting an activity program or if you want to make changes to your current activity program, turn the page. We're ready if you are!

Table 3   Action-Oriented Versus Staged Approach to Change

Action-oriented approach	Staged approach
Change is an either–or event.	Change is a fluid process.
Change is a quick fix.	Change takes time and effort.
Change is simple.	Change is complex but possible.
People are either ready to change or not.	People move through stages of readiness to change.
If you lapse, you must start all over.	If you lapse, you can get back on track. You won't go all the way back to your old habits.
If you have failed in the past, you are likely to fail again.	If you lapse, you can learn from your experience and try again. You are likely to be successful the next time you try.

What's in It for You?

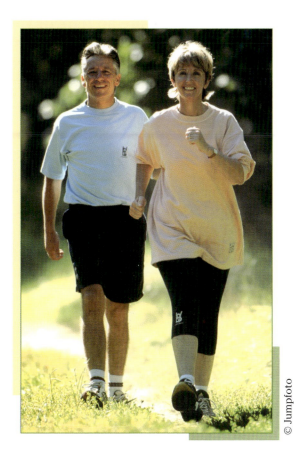

© Jumpfoto

In This Chapter

❏ Determine your stage of readiness to increase your activity.

❏ Learn specific ways that being physically active benefits older adults.

❏ Understand the risks of being physically active.

❏ Know whether you need to see your doctor before getting started.

❏ Plan how to talk with your doctor about physical activity.

❏ Think about why you might need to become more physically active.

The purpose of *Fitness After 50* is to help you be physically active for the rest of your life. Think of this goal as a journey, not a destination. On your journey to lifelong physical activity, you should know your starting point or current activity level. You can't measure your progress and celebrate your successes if you don't know where you started and how far you have come.

The Readiness to Change Questionnaire in action box 1.1 is one way to mark your starting point. Are you active now? How active have you been in the past and for how long? Do you intend to increase your physical activity level in the near future? There are no right or wrong answers. Your responses will suggest that you are in one of the five stages of readiness for changing your physical activity habits. Knowing your stage of readiness will help you focus on skills and strategies that will keep you moving forward. We will encourage you to repeat the questionnaire several times as you progress through this book.

Action Box 1.1: Readiness to Change Questionnaire

1. Are you accumulating at least 30 minutes of **moderate-intensity*** physical activity on **most (five or more) days of the week?**

    If no, go to #2.

    If yes, go to #7.

2. Are you accumulating at least **30** minutes of moderate-intensity physical activity **at least one day per week?**

    If no, go to #3.

    If yes, go to #6.

3. Do you intend to increase your physical activity?

    If no, go to #4.

    If yes, go to #5.

4. If you're not even thinking about it, **you are in the precontemplation stage.**

5. If you're giving it a thought now and then but are not doing it, **you are in the contemplation stage.**

6. If you're doing physical activity irregularly, **you are in the preparation stage.**

7. Have you been doing this regularly for the last six months?

    If no, go to #8.

    If yes, go to #9.

8. If you're doing this consistently but for less than six months, **you are in the action stage.**

9. If you've maintained the new habit for six months or more, **you are in the maintenance stage.**

* Moderate-intensity physical activities are equal in effort to a brisk walk, walking a mile (1.6 kilometers) in 15 to 20 minutes. Here are examples of other moderate-intensity activities:

Bicycling (10-12 mph or 16-19 kph), dancing, gardening and yard work, golfing (without a cart), hiking, playing actively with children, raking leaves, vacuuming a carpet, playing volleyball, washing and waxing a car

Adapted, by permission, from S. Blair, A. Dunn, B. Marcus, R. Carpenter, and P. Jaret, 2001, *Active living every day* (Champaign, IL: Human Kinetics), 9.

Knowing what stage you are in can guide you in using the right skills to help you get started or maintain your current level of physical activity. For instance, if you are in an early stage—just thinking about being active—you might need to learn more about physical activity and what it can do for you. But if you're already very active, you might be interested in finding ways to add variety or deal with the times when you have difficulty being active. *Fitness After 50* is tailored for you! See table 1.1 for ideas on where to find the information you need in this book. We encourage you to start with chapter 1 and work your way through the entire book, but table 1.1 highlights the parts of the book that might be of most interest to you.

Table 1.1   How to Find What You Need

Your stage of readiness to change (from the Readiness to Change Questionnaire in action box 1.1)	Where to look in *Fitness After 50*
Precontemplation	Not sure if physical activity is for you? Start with chapters 1 to 3.
Contemplation	Wondering why or how to get started? See chapters 1 to 4.
Preparation	Start with chapter 1, but you'll probably find chapters 4 to 8 useful.
Action	Start with chapter 1. Chapters 6 to 10 will help you refine your plans. Also see chapter 12 about anticipating and preventing lapses, which is especially important when getting started.
Maintenance	Wanting to plan a balanced program? See chapters 6 to 10. Wanting to anticipate and prevent lapses? See chapter 11. Wanting to influence others? See chapter 12.

No matter where you are starting in your journey to become more physically active, you should remind yourself of the benefits. You may have picked up this book on a whim and not be sure that physical activity is for you. On the other hand, you might be very active and looking for new and different ways to keep fit. Or maybe you've been injured or have a health problem and wonder if physical activity can still be part of your life as you get older. In most cases, physical activity can and should be part of your daily life. The benefits, especially for people over age 50, are too impressive to ignore.

Do You Know?

By age 70, about 30 percent of men and almost 40 percent of women are inactive. Overall, about 25 percent of adults are inactive, and the proportion who are inactive increases with age. An alarming 31 percent of children don't get as much exercise as they need (Centers for Disease Control and Prevention 2004).

How Did Society Become So Inactive?

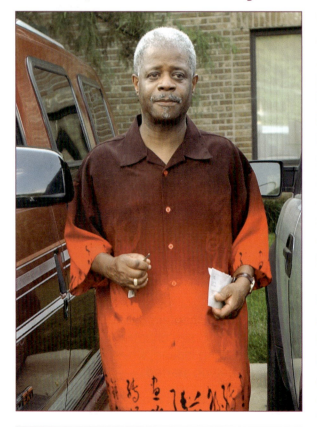

Consider parking and walking into the building instead of using drive-up windows.

Before we review the many benefits of physical activity, let's consider how our activity patterns have changed over the years. Physical activity levels of people in the industrialized countries have declined throughout the past 100 years. Physical activity has been engineered out of daily life. The increase in work hours and decline in leisure time have combined to produce an inactive lifestyle for many people.

The decline was faster during the period of economic growth after World War II. The use of labor-saving devices at work, at home, and during leisure time has continued to decrease the amount of energy needed for some tasks. You probably don't remember the first time you changed TV channels with a remote, used the drive-through lane at the bank, or paid at the pump. These actions are now routine for many of us. You can now spend the great majority of your waking hours sitting or engaged in only minimal movement. Indeed, the greatest financial and professional rewards may come to those who spend most of their time sitting at a desk.

Examples of how physical activity has been engineered from daily life are shown in table 1.2. With a little thought you can come up with many more activity choices that you must make each day. The calorie estimates in the examples are for a person weighing 150 to 160 pounds (68 to 72 kilograms). Over the course of one month, you would burn much more energy by doing tasks the active way rather than by taking the less active approach. Always taking the active approach could amount to a loss of 20 pounds (about 8 kilograms) or more in a year, if you kept your eating habits the same. None of these active ways of doing tasks is by itself significant, but collectively they can cause a drastic increase in overall physical activity for many people. Which of the ways to burn extra energy can you add to your daily life?

Table 1.2   How Do You Perform These Daily Tasks?

Do you look for ways to avoid activity?	Calories (kilojoules) burned	Do you look for ways to burn extra calories?	Calories (kilojoules) burned
Using the remote to change TV channels from your recliner	<1 (<4.2)	Getting up and changing the TV channel (total of 5 minutes per day)	3 (12.5)
Answering the phone with a nearby cordless phone; talking 30 minutes while reclining	4 (16.7)	Getting up and answering the phone and then standing during three 10-minute conversations	20 (83.6)
Using a garage door opener from the car	<1 (<4.2)	Opening the garage door twice a day	2-3 (8.4-12.5)
Hiring someone else to clean the house and do the ironing	0 (0)	30 minutes of vacuuming and 30 minutes of ironing once a week	152 (635.4)
Waiting 30 minutes for pizza delivery	15 (62.7)	30 minutes of cooking	25 (104.5)
Driving to the car wash, getting out, paying, and getting back in the car	18 (75.2)	Washing and waxing the car (60 minutes per month)	300 (1,254)
Letting the dog out the back door	2 (8.4)	Walking the dog for 30 minutes a day	125 (522.5)

(continued)

Table 1.2 *Continued*

Do you look for ways to avoid activity?	Calories (kilojoules) burned	Do you look for ways to burn extra calories?	Calories (kilojoules) burned
Driving a car to work for 40 minutes and then walking 5 minutes from the parking lot to the building	22 (92)	Walking 20 minutes to the bus stop, riding 30 minutes, and then walking 5 minutes to work	60 (250.8)
E-mailing a coworker a message (twice daily) for 4 minutes	2-3 (8.4-12.5)	Walking for 1 minute and talking with a coworker while standing for 3 minutes twice a day	6 (25)
Taking the elevator	<1 (<4.2)	Climbing one flight of stairs, three times a day	15 (62.7)
Internet shopping for an hour	30 (125.4)	Walking briskly at a mall or shopping center for an hour once a month (240 calories); strolling for an hour (145 calories)	145-240 (606-1,003)
Sitting in the car at a drive-up window three times per week for a total of 30 minutes	15 (62.7)	Parking next to the door of a restaurant, bank, dry cleaner, or convenience store and going into the building three times per week for a total of 30 minutes	70 (292.6)

Adapted from material featured in *The Dallas Morning News,* August 30, 1999.

Health Benefits of Physical Activity

Physicians and philosophers in ancient China and Greece wrote about the health benefits of regular physical activity, but until recently we really didn't know just how important regular activity is in preserving health and function. Scientific study of the effects of regular physical activity on health did not begin in earnest until the mid-1950s. Over the past 50 years, thousands of research studies published in the scientific literature have proved the numerous benefits of being active. See the impressive list of benefits outlined in table 1.3. Which of these benefits are important to you now? Which will be important to you as you get older? People have often said that if the benefits of physical activity could be put in a pill, it would be the next blockbuster drug.

Table 1.3   Health Benefits of Regular Physical Activity

Increasing physical activity improves . . .	Increasing physical activity decreases . . .
Longevity	Risk of heart attack
Flexibility	Risk of stroke
Function and independent living	Risk of developing type 2 diabetes
Bone strength	Risk of some cancers
Restful sleep	Risk of fractures
Weight control	Depression
Well-being	Obesity
	Risk of memory loss and dementia
	Risk of gall bladder disease

Do You Know?

People 50 and over know the benefits of physical activity. Here's how physically active respondents to an AARP survey ranked the benefits:

Improves overall health	83%
More energy	69%
Prevents disease	67%
Reduces stress	60%
Controls weight	60%
Looking good	48%
Socializing with others	34%
Better sex	28%

Data from AARP 2002.

So, are you beginning to see what's in it for you? Physical activity is one of the most important things you can do for your health. But that seems too general and too vague. You'd probably like detailed guidance and direction. Let's look at some of the specific benefits of regular physical activity.

■ **Delays death and extends life.** If you are fit and active, you are likely to live longer than you will if you are unfit and inactive. You need to be only moderately fit to get a health benefit (figure 1.1). Taking just three

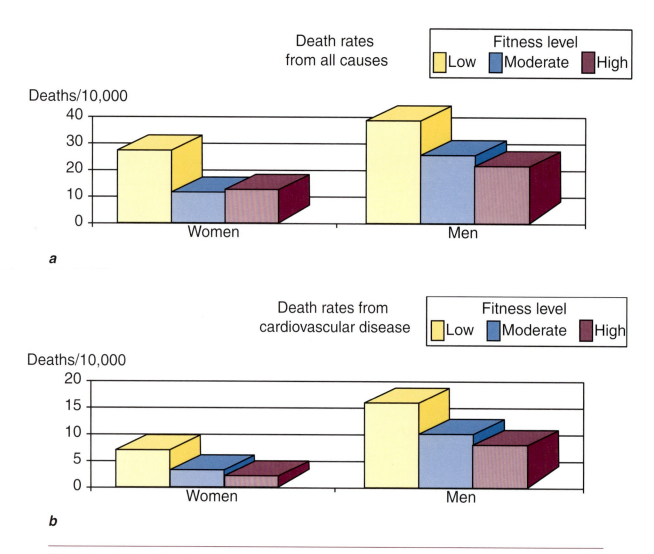

10-minute walks a day on at least five days of the week is enough for you to be moderately fit.

■ **Reduces risk of type 2 diabetes.** Type 2 diabetes is an important risk factor for heart attacks and strokes, and can lead to other serious health problems, including blindness and kidney failure. People who are regularly active and maintain normal weight rarely develop type 2 diabetes. If you already have type 2 diabetes, regular physical activity can help you keep your blood glucose level under control and reduce your risk of dying.

■ **Reduces risk of some cancers.** Lack of physical activity is now recognized as an important risk factor for some cancers. Evidence is strong that inactivity contributes to colon cancer. It is also likely that physical inactivity increases the risk of breast cancer, and it may increase risk of lung cancer and prostate cancer. All of these are the most common and feared cancers. Scientists are also learning that being active provides many benefits during cancer treatment.

■ **Keeps bones strong.** Both women and men can preserve bone as they age by being physically active, even if they have been inactive in the past. Any weight-bearing activity, such as walking, lifting weights, or digging in the

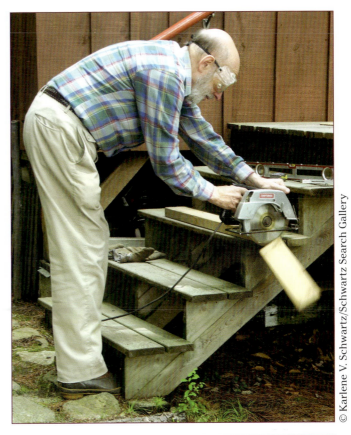

Becoming physically active will help you be able to do the things you like to do (and need to do) for a long time to come.

garden, is beneficial. The benefit of physical activity extends beyond the direct effect on the bones. For example, if you're active, you may have better coordination and balance and be less likely to fall. (Falls are the major cause of hip fractures.) Having strong muscles also means that you are less likely to fall. In addition, an active person who is strong will have large muscles that may provide some padding and protection against a fracture, even if a fall occurs.

■ **Preserves function and independence.** Much of the frailty in older people is due to decades of physical inactivity. Inactivity over the years causes a decline in both muscle fitness and aerobic fitness. When you don't have enough muscle fitness and aerobic fitness to perform the daily tasks of life, you have lost functional fitness—the ability to perform daily tasks such as bathing, cooking, and turning a key. See action box 1.2 for a list of activities of daily living. Think about what you want to be able to do for yourself now and in the future.

■ **Relieves joint pain and stiffness.** If you have osteoarthritis, don't be afraid to participate in regular moderate physical activity, which can improve your fitness and health and reduce joint pain and stiffness. Look

Action Box 1.2: Activities of Daily Living—What Do You Want to Be Able to Do for Yourself?

Check the activities of daily living that you want to be able to do when you are older.

_____ Moderate recreational activities—leisure bicycling, fishing, ballroom dancing

_____ Strenuous recreational activities—jogging, cross-country skiing, tennis, team sports

_____ Light household activities—cooking, ironing, painting inside

_____ Moderate household activities—general carpentry, cleaning, raking

_____ Strenuous household activities—digging in the garden, mowing, shoveling snow

_____ Moderate personal care activities—bathing, going to the toilet, dressing, getting in and out of bed, a chair, and the bathtub

_____ Activities requiring dexterity—writing, turning a key, buttoning

at the following list of the many reasons to become more physically active, especially if you already have osteoarthritis.

Easier movement

Stronger muscles for more stable joints

Decreased pain

Decreased medication use

Weight control

Stronger heart and better endurance

Better posture and physical appearance

Better sleep

Improved sense of well-being

■ **Improves mood and memory.** Several studies show improvement in overall feelings of general well-being in people who change from inactive to active ways of life, mostly because activity reduces feelings of tension and anxiety. Activity also may help reduce depression. Many psychologists and psychiatrists use physical activity to treat people with clinical anxiety

Myth Buster

Myth: Exercising arthritic joints, such as knees and hips, increases damage to cartilage and bone.

Fact: Rest and inactivity are the worst things that you can do if you have arthritis. Physical activity, in fact, is the mainstay of care. Physical activity helps joints work better, strengthens the supportive tissues around the joints, relieves stiffness, and makes it easier to move and get around. At the same time, increased physical activity may improve overall health by reducing blood pressure, cholesterol, and the risk of developing type 2 diabetes. Regular physical activity, such as walking or swimming, provides important health benefits for people with arthritis. If you have arthritis, consult your doctor about increasing your physical activity.

and depression. We are not yet certain that physical activity plays a role in preventing loss of memory and other mental functions. But a recent study showed that people 65 years of age and older who were physically active had a 31 percent lower risk of developing Alzheimer's disease when compared with their peers who were inactive (Lindsay et al. 2002).

■ **Helps control weight.** Has it been a struggle for you to control your weight as you have gotten older? Weight control is a common problem. You may have noticed that the number of people—both adults and children—who are overweight is greater than it was in the past. People who are overweight are more likely to develop high blood pressure, heart disease, stroke, type 2 diabetes, and some types of cancer. Being overweight is also a problem for people with arthritis in their knees. Emotional and social issues are also associated with being overweight. No one wants to be fat! Here's the inside information on how physical activity affects weight control.

   ■ **Lose modest amounts of weight:** The role of activity in losing weight is relatively modest. Physical activity is beneficial, but it does not produce large weight loss. Burning a large amount of energy by physical activity is difficult, especially for people who are overweight, inactive, and unfit to begin with. But that doesn't mean you shouldn't include physical activity in your weight loss program. You just shouldn't expect activity to cause you to lose a lot of weight quickly. There are other important reasons to be physically active.

   ■ **Keep weight off after you've lost it:** Who is most likely to keep weight off over the long term? People who have lost a large amount of weight and have kept it off for years are physically active. The majority of these successful weight maintainers are physically active for 60 to 80 minutes per day. If you want to be successful in controlling your weight for the rest of your life, learn how to increase your activity and maintain it over the long term.

■ **Prevent weight gain in the first place:** People who are inactive and stay that way over time gain more weight than do those who take up regular physical activity. According to one study, if you are inactive but become physically active, you reduce your chances of gaining 20 pounds (9 kilograms) in the next five years by about 60 percent. So, if you want to avoid overweight and obesity in the first place, changing from an inactive to an active way of life is a good plan.

■ **Enjoy the health benefits at any weight:** Regular physical activity and moderate to high levels of aerobic fitness provide health benefits to people of all sizes and shapes. In other words, regular physical activity may not give you a slender figure that is the envy of all your friends, but it will improve your health. Focus on being active and getting fit. As shown in figure 1.2, physical activity and fitness will benefit your health and extend your life even if you are overweight.

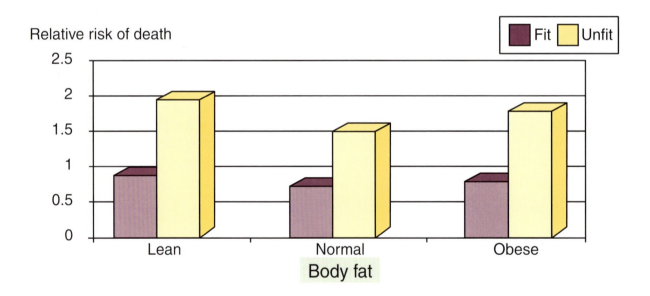

■ **Figure 1.2**   Fitness, fatness, and the risk of death (Lee, Blair, and Jackson 1999). Lean men were defined as those with less than 17 percent body fat. Normal men had 17 to 24.9 percent body fat. Obese men had 25 percent or greater body fat. Men also were classified as fit or unfit, based on their performance on a maximal exercise test on a treadmill. The least fit 20 percent of men were classified as unfit, and all the rest were classified as fit. In these calculations, the lean and fit men are the reference group and are assigned a risk of death of 1.0. The risk of dying for all other groups is expressed relative to that group. Therefore, if a group is at 2.0, that means their risk of dying is double that of the reference group.

Risks of Physical Activity

Maybe you've heard a story of a person who collapsed while walking on a treadmill at the gym. You may know someone who decided to get fit and then twisted an ankle. Are these rare events, or are they something that you should be concerned about?

For most people, the risks of most kinds of physical activity are low. The risks of being inactive are 100 percent. Two categories of risks are associated with physical activity:

- The risk of heart attack or sudden death during activity
- The risk of injury to bones, joints, ligaments, or muscles

Heart Attack or Sudden Death

Death resulting from physical activity is rare, but when someone dies of a heart attack during a recreational or sporting activity, the event receives much more attention and publicity than the same event that occurs to someone who is sitting at a desk or watching television. A recent study evaluated deaths in a large chain of fitness centers (Franklin et al. 2005). There were only 71 deaths (61 in men and 10 in women) in 2.9 million members over a two-year period. This means that there was only 1 death per 82,000 members or 1 death per every 2.57 million exercise sessions. Obviously, the risk of being physically active is very low.

Of course, you should never ignore pain, pressure, or a sense of fullness in your chest that occurs with physical activity. Be especially alert to pain or pressure coming from the jaw, shoulder, or arm. See table 1.4 for normal and abnormal symptoms during physical activity. If you notice abnormal

Table 1.4   Symptoms During Physical Activity

What is normal	What is not normal
Faster pulse	Heaviness in your chest (angina)
A few skipped heart beats	Chest pain, pain in the arm, neck, or jaw
Breathing deeply	Irregular heartbeats
Breathing faster	Extreme breathlessness
Sweating	Wheezing, not being able to catch your breath
	Light-headedness
	Nausea
	Extreme fatigue
	Numbness
	Pain of any kind

symptoms when you are physically active, especially if they go away when you stop and rest, call your doctor immediately. If these symptoms are quite noticeable and persist, you should call for emergency help. Many people assume that these symptoms are due to indigestion and they ignore them. The problem may well be a minor one, but being cautious is better than being sorry. If the pain is due to coronary artery disease, a condition that disrupts blood flow to the heart, you may be having a heart attack, in which case minutes count. The sooner you get medical attention, the less damage to your heart and the fewer consequences.

Myth Buster

Myth: Physical activity can cause a heart attack and sudden death.

Fact: Although a person who participates in regular physical activity has a greater risk of dying while active than while inactive, the regularly active person has a much lower overall risk of heart attack or sudden death than does a person who is very inactive. A physically active person is more likely to have a heart attack during heavy physical exertion than he or she is when not exercising, but a physically inactive person is 50 times more likely than an active person is to have a heart attack during physical activity.

Research News You Can Use

Question: How risky is physical activity for people in a cardiac rehabilitation program?

Answer: Not very risky! Only three sudden cardiac deaths occurred in 51,303 cardiac patients in 167 rehabilitation programs (Franklin et al. 1998). They participated in more than 2.3 million hours of exercise over a 5-year period. At this rate, a person would have to go to the rehabilitation program three times a week for more than 5,000 years before dying suddenly during exercise.

How you can use this news: You can feel confident that the moderate level of physical activity recommended in this book is safe for almost everyone, even people with heart disease.

Minor Aches and Pains

Muscle soreness and stiffness are common when you start a physical activity program or resume activity after a long layoff. These effects are not permanent or serious injuries but rather natural reactions to using muscles that you haven't been using regularly. You can expect to feel some soreness when you first start or when you change or increase your activity. The soreness will be temporary and will pass as you become active more regularly.

You also can strain muscles, tendons, or ligaments during activity. These types of overuse injuries come from long sessions of physical activity or from sudden overstretching of muscles or joints. The risk of these injuries increases with the intensity of the activity. See chapter 11 for more information on what to do if you think you've strained something.

The most serious injuries are sprains, fractures, torn ligaments, and torn muscles. Sprains commonly occur in the ankle, knee, and shoulder. Severe sprains or tears of the ligaments result from injuries in which too much force or torque is applied at the joint. Broken bones generally occur from falling and usually are associated with activities such as skating or snow skiing, which can result in high-impact falls. On rare occasions, physical activity can cause a stress fracture—a minute crack in a bone. These fractures occur from repetitive pounding on a weak area of the bone, usually in the foot, lower leg, or hip. The major symptom of a stress fracture is persistent pain. A stress fracture is difficult to diagnose because it doesn't show up on a standard X-ray. Diagnosis requires an MRI or bone scan.

Although injuries to the muscles, joints, and bones are likely to increase with age, you can do several things to protect against them. For example, if you've been walking a little, now is not the time to try to run three miles. You need to work up to such activities gradually and at your own pace. Remember that you don't need to do strenuous activity to reap most health benefits. You need not go all out if you're just starting to become physically active. You can also protect against sprains, strains, and other injuries by using proper technique and equipment. In later chapters we'll help you learn more about planning safe and effective fitness programs. Furthermore, the type and amount of activity recommended in this book generally have low risk for injury.

Should You See Your Doctor?

If you are in good health and plan a gradual increase in moderate activities, such as walking, you are not likely to need to see your doctor. Take a few minutes right now to complete the PAR-Q (Physical Activity Readiness Questionnaire) in action box 1.3. The PAR-Q, developed by Canadian public health and exercise experts, helps determine whether you may benefit from a medical exam before increasing your activity. The PAR-Q is one of several popular screening tools used by fitness professionals and fitness centers to screen clients and members.

Physical Activity Readiness
Questionnaire - PAR-Q
(revised 2002)

PAR-Q & YOU
(A Questionnaire for People Aged 15 to 69)

Regular physical activity is fun and healthy, and increasingly more people are starting to become more active every day. Being more active is very safe for most people. However, some people should check with their doctor before they start becoming much more physically active.

If you are planning to become much more physically active than you are now, start by answering the seven questions in the box below. If you are between the ages of 15 and 69, the PAR-Q will tell you if you should check with your doctor before you start. If you are over 69 years of age, and you are not used to being very active, check with your doctor.

Common sense is your best guide when you answer these questions. Please read the questions carefully and answer each one honestly: check YES or NO.

YES	NO	
❑	❑	1. Has your doctor ever said that you have a heart condition <u>and</u> that you should only do physical activity recommended by a doctor?
❑	❑	2. Do you feel pain in your chest when you do physical activity?
❑	❑	3. In the past month, have you had chest pain when you were not doing physical activity?
❑	❑	4. Do you lose your balance because of dizziness or do you ever lose consciousness?
❑	❑	5. Do you have a bone or joint problem (for example, back, knee or hip) that could be made worse by a change in your physical activity?
❑	❑	6. Is your doctor currently prescribing drugs (for example, water pills) for your blood pressure or heart condition?
❑	❑	7. Do you know of <u>any other reason</u> why you should not do physical activity?

If

you

answered

YES to one or more questions

Talk with your doctor by phone or in person BEFORE you start becoming much more physically active or BEFORE you have a fitness appraisal. Tell your doctor about the PAR-Q and which questions you answered YES.

- You may be able to do any activity you want — as long as you start slowly and build up gradually. Or, you may need to restrict your activities to those which are safe for you. Talk with your doctor about the kinds of activities you wish to participate in and follow his/her advice.
- Find out which community programs are safe and helpful for you.

NO to all questions

If you answered NO honestly to <u>all</u> PAR-Q questions, you can be reasonably sure that you can:

- start becoming much more physically active – begin slowly and build up gradually. This is the safest and easiest way to go.
- take part in a fitness appraisal – this is an excellent way to determine your basic fitness so that you can plan the best way for you to live actively. It is also highly recommended that you have your blood pressure evaluated. If your reading is over 144/94, talk with your doctor before you start becoming much more physically active.

DELAY BECOMING MUCH MORE ACTIVE:

- if you are not feeling well because of a temporary illness such as a cold or a fever – wait until you feel better; or
- if you are or may be pregnant – talk to your doctor before you start becoming more active.

PLEASE NOTE: If your health changes so that you then answer YES to any of the above questions, tell your fitness or health professional. Ask whether you should change your physical activity plan.

Informed Use of the PAR-Q: The Canadian Society for Exercise Physiology, Health Canada, and their agents assume no liability for persons who undertake physical activity, and if in doubt after completing this questionnaire, consult your doctor prior to physical activity.

No changes permitted. You are encouraged to photocopy the PAR-Q but only if you use the entire form.

NOTE: If the PAR-Q is being given to a person before he or she participates in a physical activity program or a fitness appraisal, this section may be used for legal or administrative purposes.

"I have read, understood and completed this questionnaire. Any questions I had were answered to my full satisfaction."

NAME _____

SIGNATURE _____ DATE _____

SIGNATURE OF PARENT _____ WITNESS _____
or GUARDIAN (for participants under the age of majority)

Note: This physical activity clearance is valid for a maximum of 12 months from the date it is completed and becomes invalid if your condition changes so that you would answer YES to any of the seven questions.

© Canadian Society for Exercise Physiology

Supported by: Health   Santé
Canada   Canada

Physical Activity Readiness Questionnaire (PAR-Q) © 2002.

Reprinted with permission of the Canadian Society for Exercise Physiology, Inc.   www.csep.ca/forms.asp

If you answered "No" to all questions in the PAR-Q, you can increase your physical activity by beginning slowly and building up gradually. If at any time in the future one of your answers becomes a "Yes," see your doctor to discuss your physical activity plans.

If you answered "Yes" to one or more questions on the PAR-Q, talk with your doctor before you start becoming much more physically active or before you have a fitness appraisal.

You are probably most interested in moderate physical activity—activities that are equal in effort to a brisk walk. If you're already very active, however, you might be wanting to try vigorous activities. Vigorous physical activities make you breathe hard and sweat. Jogging is an example of a vigorous activity. If you want to exercise at a vigorous level, check with your doctor first if you

- are a man 45 or older or a woman 55 or older; or

- have two or more of the following risk factors: have a family history of heart disease, are currently a cigarette smoker, have high blood pressure, have high cholesterol, have high blood sugar, are at least 30 pounds (13.6 kilograms) overweight, or are currently not at all active; or

- have heart or blood vessel disease, diabetes, lung disease, asthma, thyroid disorders, or kidney disease (Blair 2001).

Questions for Your Doctor

Getting approval before starting is only one reason to talk with your doctor about physical activity. A second reason is to talk about the benefits of being active as you get older. Visit with your doctor about physical activity as part of your regular preventive checkups. You may want to show your doctor this book to open the discussion about physical activity. Action box 1.4 includes a list of questions that can guide your visit with your doctor about physical activity. Add your own questions and issues to the list and take it with you to your next visit. As for any visit, be prepared. Take all your medicines with you, including over-the-counter medicines and supplements.

Action Box 1.4: Questions for Your Doctor About Physical Activity

Use this list of questions to talk with your doctor about physical activity. Add other questions that are important to you in the blank spaces. Take notes as you talk with your doctor.

(continued)

Questions	Answers, notes
Is it safe for me to increase my physical activity?	
Should I avoid any types of physical activity?	
How do I know if I'm doing too much or not enough?	
What symptoms could mean trouble during physical activity?	
Do I need any tests before I increase my activity?	
Do my medications need to be changed when I increase my physical activity?	

More information about medical conditions common in people over age 50 is presented in chapter 3. You will also learn how you can adapt your activity program to meet your special needs.

Your Thoughts and Feelings About Physical Activity

So far in this chapter you have identified your stage of readiness to change your physical activity habits. You have learned about some of the specific benefits of physical activity and fitness that are important for people over age 50. You have also learned that the benefits of physical activity far outweigh the risks. Now, are you thinking seriously about increasing your activity level? When you think about changing your physical activity habits, what feelings do you have?

Rarely does anyone embrace change once and for all. Most people tend to alternate between resisting change and embracing it. Just as the payoffs of becoming more active will pull you toward your goal, unforeseen forces will pull you back to your inactive ways.

Use action box 1.5 to evaluate the positive and negative forces that pull you toward and push you away from your goal of becoming more active. Later in this book you will use this information to increase the positive forces that will help you become active and reduce the negative forces that are working against you.

Action Box 1.5:   Evaluating Positive and Negative Forces

Mark the forces that you are experiencing now. What others would you add to the list?

Advantages of remaining inactive: If I stay inactive . . .	Disadvantages of being active: If I become active . . .
__ I won't have to change any habits.	__ I could get injured.
__ My friends who are inactive won't feel intimidated.	__ I will miss watching television.
__ I won't have to put out any effort.	__ I will sweat, and I don't like that.
__ I will have no risk of failure.	__ I will have less time to spend with friends and family.

Disadvantages of remaining inactive: If I stay inactive . . .	Advantages of being active: If I become active . . .
__ My health is likely to get worse.	__ I will make new friends.
__ My endurance level will decline.	__ I will feel more confident.
__ I may lose my ability to function.	__ I will look better.
__ I may not be able to live independently.	__ I will have more energy and stamina to do the things I enjoy.

Summary

You began this chapter by completing the Readiness to Change Questionnaire. We'll remind you to repeat it in later chapters to check your progress. We also highlighted the benefits of physical activity and physical fitness for people over age 50. Are you beginning to realize that regular participation in physical activity is one of the best things that you can do for yourself and your health? Staying active and fit extends life and protects against the development of many diseases that are common in people over age 50. It also improves your quality of life, preserves function, and allows you to live independently for longer. For most of us, this last benefit is the greatest of all.

We hope that this chapter has helped you take an important first step toward becoming more active. Congratulations! You're on your way!

Chapter Checklist

Following are some ways in which you can apply what you have learned in this chapter to your daily life. Take time over the next days and weeks to put these recommendations into action.

- ❑ Consider where you are right now—your stage of readiness to change your physical activity habits. Complete the readiness questionnaire.

- ❑ Think about the health benefits of physical activity that are important to you.

- ❑ Complete the PAR-Q. Make an appointment to see your doctor if necessary.

- ❑ Consider how you think about change. Do you generally resist or embrace change? What are the positive and negative forces affecting your efforts to be active? If you feel that you are not yet ready to get started with activity, focus on starting to think about becoming more active. Thinking seriously about physical activity is the first step in getting started.

Word Search

See if you can find 10 important words from this chapter in the grid that appears below. Words appear forward and backward in rows, columns, and diagonals. The solution is shown on page 231.

```
C K Y J Z S G F J A A P I N R
W O S S E N I D A E R Q N O I
P N N F S S M J E E N N D I S
F Y P T N R N H P L K F E T K
S U U D E Y S A O G N X P C S
M T K O H M R T Y D D O E N O
H Z I M U A P E A Y D Z N U P
W O H F T C G L H G Z H D F P
S C X I E N Y G A E E Y E A N
E F O V A N Q J B T D F N Y J
M N B H T C E T A W I C C G N
V Z C F T Y R B L M O O E P U
H W P B T B V G Y L W V N N A
G K Q H F T F C O S P C W U N
G B A C T I O N R X K Y D J O
```

Action	Function	Readiness
Benefits	Independence	Risks
Change	Preparation	Stage
Contemplation		

What You Think Matters

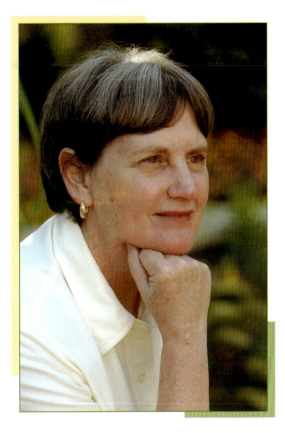

In This Chapter

- ❏ Review ways in which you have changed lifestyle habits in the past.
- ❏ Learn how what you think influences what you feel and do.
- ❏ Recognize and challenge excuses for not being active.
- ❏ Consider the advantages and disadvantages for being active that are important to you.

Almost all people know that being active is good for them. But, some people consider changing their health habits only after a dramatic event captures their attention. Consider the cases of Gary, Kathy, and Marie.

Personal Profiles

Gary, Age 50

After working for a large company for more than 20 years, Gary is excited about starting his own business. His business plan requires outside financing. A bank is interested in his concept and agrees to back his business but requires a life insurance policy as part of the security for the loan. When Gary goes for his life insurance physical, he is surprised to learn that his cholesterol is at a borderline high level, and he is moderately overweight. His doctor recommends more physical activity to reduce his risk factors and to help deal with the stress of the new business.

Kathy, Age 56

Kathy, who has been single for nearly 15 years, has finally met the man of her dreams. They are planning a small wedding next summer. Her fiancé is an avid outdoorsman. He enjoys golf, fishing, sailing, hiking, mountain biking, and traveling to exotic places. He is planning a honeymoon vacation that includes activity, adventure, and romance. With six months to get ready, Kathy is committed to improving her strength and stamina, and losing a little weight and firming up would definitely make her feel more attractive and desirable.

Marie, Age 68

Marie's sister Janet, who is three years younger, has had a stroke that leaves her partially paralyzed and facing months of physical therapy. Marie has neglected her borderline high blood pressure for years. She thinks, "If Janet can have a stroke, I could too. After all, we've got some of the same genes. I should think about making some changes before it's too late."

Physical activity could help all the people described in the personal profiles improve their health and quality of life. A life-changing event, either positive or negative, can get your attention and be a powerful stimulus for increasing your activity. Suddenly, health and lifestyle are a higher priority on your personal agenda. You begin to look seriously at the advantages of being physically active.

Let the Past Be Your Guide

You have probably made changes in your lifestyle at some time in the past. Some attempts may have been successful, whereas others likely were not. Perhaps you implemented daily flossing as part of your dental health program. Maybe you quit smoking years ago when the evidence about the health risks of smoking became too compelling to ignore. Perhaps you started getting an annual flu shot or began to read labels to know which foods to buy so that you would consume less saturated fat, cholesterol, or sodium. In any event, you probably can identify some positive health habits you have incorporated into your current lifestyle. Knowing that you have made positive changes in the past, even simple ones, should give you confidence that you can make other changes, such as increasing your physical activity.

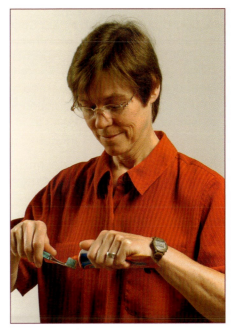

Being physically active should be a daily habit, just like brushing and flossing your teeth.

Past Successes

Take a few minutes to think about your past successes at changing a lifestyle habit. Complete action box 2.1. What worked in the past is likely to work in the future.

Action Box 2.1: Analyze Past Successes to Change

	Example	A past success	A past success
What did you change?	I decided to stop smoking.		
Why did you want to change?	I was concerned about my risk of a heart attack. Also, I wanted to be a positive role model for my children.		
How did you change? What helped you be successful?	I used nicotine replacement therapy along with a group smoking-cessation program. I didn't spend time with people who smoked.		
How many times did you try to change the habit before you were successful?	I tried to quit cold turkey four or five times over 10 years before I was able to quit for good.		

(continued)

	Example	A past success	A past success
What did you learn from your unsuccessful attempts to change?	I learned that my addiction to nicotine was stronger than I thought it was.		
What makes you continue the healthy habit?	I feel much better about my health and about myself. I can breathe easier and I don't cough as much. I feel that if I can stop smoking, I can do anything!		

Unsuccessful Attempts

Just as you can point to some successes in changing lifestyle habits, you can also identify attempts that didn't work for you. Trial and error is a good way to make a change. If you tried an approach that didn't work, you can learn from your experience, develop a new plan, and try again. Trying something different rather than repeating the same approach is the key. Unsuccessful attempts are learning opportunities. Review unsuccessful attempts to change your lifestyle by completing action box 2.2.

Action Box 2.2: Analyze Unsuccessful Attempts to Change

	Example	An unsuccessful attempt	An unsuccessful attempt
What did you want to change?	I wanted to increase my muscle strength.		
Why?	I wanted to look more fit and trim.		
What were your reasons for not changing?	I didn't like going to the fitness center to use the machines. I felt intimidated by the bodybuilders.		

	Example	An unsuccessful attempt	An unsuccessful attempt
What resistance did you face from yourself and others?	Strength building required a lot more concentration and work than I expected.		
What techniques did you use to try to change?	I hired a personal trainer to get started, but after the sessions ended, I didn't continue on my own.		
Were you successful for a short period?	I was successful for about three weeks.		
What made you stop trying?	I didn't enjoy it and didn't see results.		
What could you do differently in the future?	I might look for a program that I could do at home on my own.		

By completing the analyses of your past attempts (what worked and what didn't), you've taken an important step toward increasing your physical activity. In the examples, an organized group class helped the person successfully stop smoking. It's not surprising, then, that lack of continued support may have been a factor in not staying with the weight-training program. For this person, having a friend as a workout partner or spotter may have helped him or her stay with the strength-building program long enough to see results. You will learn strategies for getting the support of others in later chapters of this book.

Change Your Thinking

Most people believe that a particular event or situation causes their feelings and actions at any given point in time. Consider example #1. Your walking partner relocates to another area for the winter (point A). Because your partner is unavailable, you give up your walking program (point C).

But between point A and point C, something else happens: At point B, you think. The thoughts that you have are called inner dialogues. The thinking

Example #1

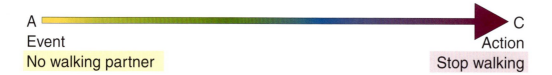

A ──────────────────────────────► C
Event   Action
No walking partner   Stop walking

that you do at point B can be rational or irrational. Many of us think irrationally at least some of the time. Some common irrational ideas are listed in action box 2.3. Do any of them describe your ways of thinking?

Consider example #2. Because your walking partner is out of town for several months, you think that it's not safe to walk because you'll be walking alone (point B). You feel discouraged and automatically decide to give up your walking program (point C).

Example #2

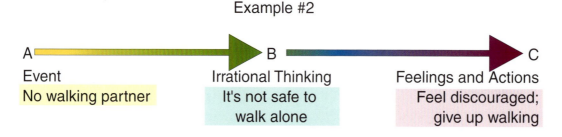

A ──────────────► B ──────────────► C
Event   Irrational Thinking   Feelings and Actions
No walking partner   It's not safe to   Feel discouraged;
                     walk alone   give up walking

Irrational thinking is illogical and self-defeating, and keeps you from attaining your goal. In contrast, rational thinking is reasonable and realistic. Rational thinking does not automatically reject negative thoughts or simply substitute positive thinking. In fact, a negative thought may be accurate and a positive thought may be inaccurate. Thinking rationally means asking if a thought is rational, and if it is, acting accordingly. If the thought is irrational, then you should replace it with a rational thought so that rational feelings and actions follow.

You can change your thoughts. Changing your thoughts is important because you are going to take your own advice. You can learn to be your own counselor or trainer.

Consider example #3. At point B ask, "Is this a rational assessment of the situation?" Although it may be true that walking alone when it is dark or in certain places may not be safe, it is not true that you can't be physically active while your partner is out of town. Instead of an irrational thought

Example #3

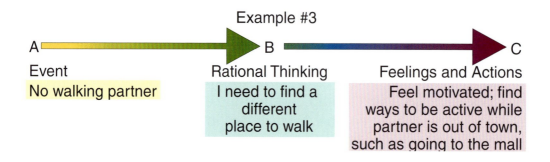

A ──────────────► B ──────────────► C
Event   Rational Thinking   Feelings and Actions
No walking partner   I need to find a   Feel motivated; find
                     different   ways to be active while
                     place to walk   partner is out of town,
                                          such as going to the mall

at point B, you could say to yourself, "I may need to find a different place or time to walk," or "I should ask someone else to walk with me." Changing your thoughts at point B will change how you feel and what you do at point C.

Action Box 2.3:   Common Irrational Ideas

Everyone thinks irrationally from time to time. Here are some common irrational ideas that may underlie your thoughts. Although each is stated in the most extreme case, you can see how each idea could influence your ability to be active. The first four ideas are the most important and most common (Ellis 1973).

Approval—You feel that you must have approval almost all the time from the people who are important to you. For example, would you be concerned that some of your friends who are inactive may not approve of your active lifestyle?

Perfectionism—You must prove yourself thoroughly competent. You feel that you must have real competence or talent at something before you will participate. For example, would you resist playing golf or tennis because you might not be able to play as well as others?

Demanding—You view life as awful, terrible, or horrible when people or things do not go easily for you. For example, would you give up a new activity because the first time you tried it you got a little stiff and sore?

Blaming—You consider people who harm you or treat you unkindly as generally bad people. You blame them for your actions. For example, would you blame others for keeping you from being active?

Irresponsibility—You find it easier to avoid facing many of the difficulties of life rather than taking responsibility for them. For example, do you make excuses about why you can't be active?

Inertia—You can be happy by doing nothing, passively "enjoying yourself." For example, would you rather stay inactive than get the benefits of physical activity?

Do any of these apply to you? Write about how a thought or feeling has influenced your physical activity in the past.

_____

_____

_____

_____

_____

Stop and Think

Irrational beliefs about physical activity may pop into your head from time to time. But you can learn to change your thoughts (Ellis 1974). Stop, analyze your thoughts (inner dialogues), and substitute a more rational, accurate thought, if necessary, before you act. You can stop the process of automatic thinking and change your feelings and actions. Practice analyzing and changing thoughts by completing action box 2.4. You may have already had some of these thoughts in the past. Try to be more aware of how your thinking affects your actions in the next week.

Action Box 2.4: Substitute Rational for Irrational Thoughts

Analyze each irrational thought. Ask yourself, "Is it accurate and reasonable?" Change the thought to a more rational belief.
Example:

Irrational thought: Exercise is for athletes, and I'm not athletic.	
Ask yourself, "Is this thought accurate and reasonable?"	No. I know several people just like me who aren't athletes but are physically active. They participate in noncompetitive activities such as walking and seem to enjoy them.
Change the thought to a more rational belief.	I may not be an athlete, but I can participate in physical activity, have fun, and obtain many health benefits.

Inaccurate, irrational, negative thoughts	Accurate, rational, positive thoughts
I have never been active. Is this thought accurate and reasonable? Explain.	
In the right-hand column, write an accurate thought to replace this one.	
My friends who are inactive won't approve of my activity. Is this thought accurate and reasonable? Explain.	
In the right-hand column, write an accurate thought to replace this one.	

Recognize and Challenge Excuses

Excuses are a type of irrational thought that you can believe and accept without even thinking. Excuses can blind you to options and prevent problem solving. Here are two of the most common excuses for not being active that we've heard from people over age 50, followed by constructive responses. Do any of these comments sound like something you might say?

Excuse: "I'm too old to be active."

Constructive response: You're never too old to be active. People as old as 90 or 100 years of age can increase their strength and aerobic fitness and therefore improve their ability to perform daily tasks.

Excuse: "I think exercise is boring. I don't think I'd enjoy it."

Constructive response: What types of physical activity or exercise have you tried in the past? You can be physically active in many ways without doing structured exercise. Maybe having a partner or being part of a group is key to your enjoyment. See chapter 8 for ways to make physical activity fun.

The excuses of others may be easier to identify than your own. One way to learn to be aware of your own excuses is to listen for "If only . . . " statements and "Yes, but . . ." responses. Complete action box 2.5. You may be surprised at how often you hear these kinds of statements.

Action Box 2.5:   What's the Excuse?

Part 1. Constructive Responses

For each of the "If only . . . " statements that you or someone else might use to avoid being active, create a new, constructive response. Add an "If only . . ." statement of your own and then reframe your response.

Excuse	Constructive response
Example: "If only I weren't so tired at the end of the day, I'd feel like exercising."	"Regular physical activity can relieve stress and make me feel more energetic at the end of the day."
"If only I didn't have to watch my grandchildren, I could be more active."	
"If only I could afford to go to a health club, I could be more active."	
"If only I didn't have arthritis."	
"If only . . ."	

(continued)

Part 2. "Yes, but" Excuses

Following are several possible solutions to common problems in increasing your physical activity. Play the devil's advocate. Write a "Yes, but . . ." excuse that you have used before or have heard someone else use. This activity will help you be more aware of your "Yes, but . . . ." excuses.

Solution	Excuse
Example: If you go for a walk first thing in the morning, nothing can prevent you from being active that day.	"Yes, but I must prepare breakfast for my husband in the morning, and I wouldn't have time to walk."
An easy way to increase your physical activity is to park your car farther from the building and walk the extra distance.	"Yes, but . . ."
If you work out with a video at home, you can save money by not paying for a fitness center membership.	"Yes, but . . ."
If you walk to lunch, you can get an extra 15 minutes of physical activity.	"Yes, but . . ."

Are You Ready?

In chapter 1 you had an opportunity to complete a questionnaire to determine your stage of readiness for physical activity. Another way to see where you are in your journey to lifelong activity is to consider the advantages and disadvantages of increasing your physical activity that are important to you now. You can use the advantages that are most important to you to help you keep a positive attitude and stay motivated.

Weigh Your Pros and Cons

Complete action box 2.6 to weigh your pros (advantages or benefits) and cons (disadvantages or barriers). If you are just starting to think about starting to be active, your score for cons will be higher than your score for pros. You probably still find more reasons

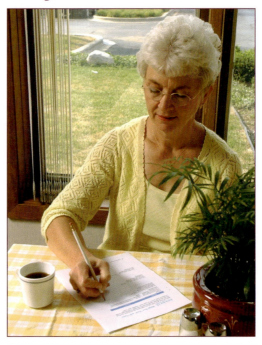

Take the time to consider the advantages and disadvantages of physical activity. As your list of pros grows, you'll be more likely to stay physically active.

for staying inactive than for being active. If you are active from time to time, but not on most days, your score for pros and cons is probably about equal. When your score for pros outweighs your score for cons, you are ready to be active regularly. If you have been active regularly for quite a while, your list of advantages is long and it will continue to grow. Your list of cons may have nearly disappeared. The longer that you are active, the more advantages and fewer disadvantages you will see for activity.

As you progress through this book, you will learn ways to increase your pros and eliminate your cons. Repeating this activity every few months will help you measure your progress.

Action Box 2.6: Weigh Your Pros and Cons

Mark the pros and cons that are important to you now. For those that are very important, place two marks in the blank. Count the total number of marks in each column. Do your pros outweigh your cons?

Advantages, or pros, for physical activity	Disadvantages, or cons, for physical activity
_____ I enjoy being physically active.	_____ I'm too tired to be active.
_____ I feel better when I am active.	_____ I'm too old to be active.
_____ Being active makes me feel young.	_____ I'll appear foolish.
_____ Physical activity reduces my risk of heart attack, stroke, and even some cancers.	_____ None of my friends are active.
	_____ I could get hurt.
_____ Physical activity helps control my blood pressure, cholesterol, and tri-glycerides.	_____ I don't like to sweat.
	_____ My allergies prevent me from being outdoors.
_____ Being active helps prevent type 2 diabetes.	_____ I just don't like physical activity.
_____ Being active increases longevity.	_____ I wouldn't be able to do other activities that I enjoy.
_____ Staying active will help me live independently for longer.	_____ My joints hurt when I move.
	_____ I might have a heart attack.
_____ I can sleep better when I am active.	_____ I don't have the money to join a fitness center.
_____ I am less likely to fall if I am fit.	
_____ I like looking trim and fit.	_____ I don't have a safe place to be active.

(continued)

➡ **Action Box 2.6: Weigh Your Pros and Cons** *(continued)*

Advantages, or pros, for physical activity	Disadvantages, or cons, for physical activity
_____ I feel more confident and in control of my life.	_____ I don't have the skills.
_____ Physical activity helps me manage my weight.	_____ I don't know what to do.
_____ I am able to take fewer medications.	_____ I don't want to have to leave home to do activity.
_____ My bones will be stronger if I am active.	Add your personal cons here.
_____ I will be able to do daily tasks and take care of myself.	
Add your personal pros here.	
Total for pros _____	Total for cons _____
Try to add at least one more pro to your list next week.	Try to eliminate at least one con from your list next week.

Take a Small Step

If you're already very active, that's great! Keep up the good work. Many of the exercises in this book will be useful when you need an extra boost or run into an obstacle in your activity plans.

If you are not yet doing physical activity, here's your chance to take one small step. Consider trying one of these options this week:

- Choose one time to try an active option instead of an inactive one: Take the stairs instead of the elevator for a couple of flights, park and walk instead of using a drive-through window, or pay inside instead of paying at the pump.

- Find a time when you can park far away and walk rather than choose the closest parking place.

- Take a two-minute walk. That's right. Find a couple times this week when you can get up and walk for two minutes. Notice how you feel afterward: Do you have more energy?

Summary

This chapter has given you a lot to think about related to your physical activity habits. Begin by thinking about the positive habits you have established in the past. What can you learn from your successful and unsuccessful attempts to change?

You've seen how thoughts about physical activity influence feelings and actions. If you are having negative or irrational thoughts about physical activity, you can change your thoughts. Focus on seeing more advantages than disadvantages for physical activity.

If you are not quite ready to develop your plan for how you will be active, then give yourself a little more time. But don't take too long. People who move from thinking about change to developing their plan for change in a relatively short time (less than 30 days) are much more likely to be successful long term. Try to get unstuck, out of the rut of inactivity, and in to the habit of regular activity.

Chapter Checklist

Following are some ways in which you can apply what you have learned in this chapter to your daily life. Over the next few days and weeks try to do as many of these activities as you can.

- ❏ Analyze your past attempts to change a habit. Identify strategies that were successful and those that were unsuccessful. You will use this information as you develop your plan to become more active.

- ❏ Listen to your inner dialogues. Learn to challenge your irrational thoughts and excuses and replace them with positive, rational thoughts.

- ❏ Try to identify at least one new advantage (pro) of being physically active that is important to you.

- ❏ Try to eliminate at least one disadvantage (con) of being physically active.

- ❏ If you are not currently active, take a small step to include some physical activity in your daily life. See how much better you feel.

Word Search

See if you can find 10 important words from this chapter in the grid that follows. Words appear forward and backward in rows, columns, and diagonals. The solution is shown on page 231.

```
S E K D P P B A M L C I P H E
T O X R I J I M P R J E T A Y
H M O C Q C R C G Z R Y P B E
G S L H U P L A Q F N X B I P
U Y Z L C S V F E R Y E T T H
O Z J O A C E C N N V H P S D
H L K S G N T S U I O C A W G
T H Z Z J I O Z T V S M Y O A
L E U G O L A I D R E N N I Q
S Y Q N N C S B T V J K Y Y X
M Y I N T O O A N A L Y Z E E
U S M W P T V E K K R D W D E
M B M F L C C O F U E S O L J
Z N Q G R Y S N O C D M R X K
I J E S G Q Z Z P D Z V B A N
```

Analyze	Inner dialogue	Pros
Cons	Perfectionism	Rational
Excuses	Positive	Thoughts
Habits		

What's Age Got to Do With It?

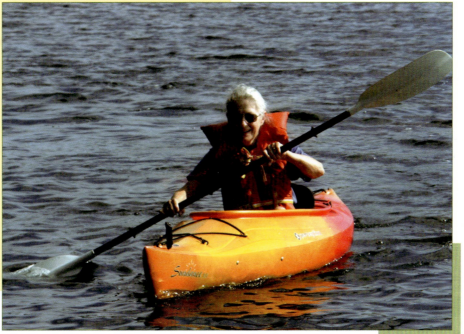

© Karlene V. Schwartz/Schwartz Search Gallery

In This Chapter

❑ Learn what to expect with aging and how getting older affects your ability to be active.

❑ Learn how physical activity helps prevent the less predictable parts of aging, such as heart disease or weight gain.

❑ Know precautions to take during activity if you have special health problems.

❑ Learn to use affirmations to help motivate yourself to be active.

❑ Keep track of your thoughts and actions related to physical activity.

Thi s could be one of the best times in your life to be physically active. You're only as old as you feel and act, and there's nothing like physical activity to keep you looking and feeling young. Moreover, physical activity helps delay or prevent many of the conditions that people commonly experience as they get older.

Your body has changed since your 20s or 30s. See action box 3.1 to check the signs of aging related to physical fitness that you are experiencing. You may be surprised to learn that some of the changes that you thought were common with age are, in fact, uncommon. Knowing what to expect as you get older makes it easier to plan a physical activity program that is safe and that will give you the results you want.

Action Box 3.1: Have You Noticed Signs of Aging?

The usual signs of aging related to physical fitness are easy to recognize, especially as you approach middle age. Do any of these describe you? Mark any that apply.

_____ Your stamina isn't what it used to be. The ability of the heart and lungs to supply the body with oxygen declines with age.

_____ You lose some flexibility. Your joints don't move as easily as they did when you were in your 20s. You notice that you are sore and stiff from your annual spring cleaning or an occasional game of softball.

_____ Muscle size and strength start to decrease after your 30s.

_____ Speed and quickness all but disappear by your early 40s. Movements that were easy to perform a few years ago seem difficult now.

_____ You put on extra weight more easily, and the weight appears in all the wrong places. Women often gain weight in the hips or thighs after childbirth and may see an increase in their waist size after menopause. Men develop beer bellies or love handles.

_____ Women may lose height in their 70s when bones lose calcium and become more brittle. Fractures are more common.

Good news: None of these changes limits function or independence, and a physically active lifestyle can delay all such changes.

Personal Profile

Ernie, Age 89

Ernie lives in a retirement community near his daughter and her family. He moved there from across the country about 15 years ago, after his wife died. He enjoys living closer to family members and watching children and grandchildren grow into adulthood. Now great-grandchildren come to visit regularly. The youngest children especially enjoy the pet rabbits that Ernie cares for every day. Ernie is undoubtedly old, but you probably wouldn't pick him as the oldest in his community. He takes a short walk each day, often stopping by neighbors' homes to say hello. He is mobile and has fewer health problems than many of the people living in his community, some of whom are 30 years younger. At his 89th birthday party, he commented, "It's great to be 89, considering the alternative!" For Ernie, there is a big difference between his health age and his real age. When asked how he has lived so long and well, he credits regular physical activity and other healthy habits.

Causes of Aging

Although recognizing the visible signs of aging is easy, the specific causes of aging remain largely unknown. Aging is a topic of hot debate among gerontologists (scientists who study aging). Experts agree, however, that aging is of two types. Aging is the result of predictable changes that occur in the body—changes that happen to everyone. Conditions such as heart disease, stroke, cancer, arthritis, and diabetes are not part of aging. These changes are less predictable and affect only certain people.

For centuries, humans have been looking for the fountain of youth. Although no magic youth potion exists, you can do many things to improve your quality of life as you age. A healthy lifestyle will add years to your life and life to your years.

Recently, a group of internationally known gerontologists (Olshansky, Hayflick, and Carnes 2002) condemned the promotion and use of antiaging medicines as worthless and without scientific merit. Instead, they endorsed efforts to practice healthy habits, such as not smoking, being physically active, and maintaining a healthy weight. Living a healthy lifestyle has been proved to prevent or delay the effects of aging. Remember, however, that nothing can stop the aging process.

Time marches on. By living an active lifestyle and staying fit, you won't prevent aging, but you can slow the rate of decline that occurs with aging. You'll also improve your health, prevent the development of health problems, and increase your chances of being healthy and independent in old age. You could be like Ernie. Age fast or age slow—it's up to you!

Changes That Occur With Age

Because the focus of this book is physical activity, we will discuss changes in the parts of the body that relate to fitness—the heart, lungs, blood vessels, muscles, bones, and joints. By themselves, the common changes that occur with age to these parts of the body usually do not cause problems. The changes can cause concern, however, if they occur faster than usual because of inactivity or disease. You will be pleased to know that regular physical activity can slow or prevent problems associated with all these changes.

Ability to Do Physical Work

Your ability to do physical work, such as washing the car or climbing stairs, depends on three things: the ability of your lungs to take in oxygen, the ability of your heart to pump oxygen-rich blood, and the ability of your muscles to use the oxygen. These functions decline moderately with age. But at any age, active people can do much more work than can people of the same age who are sedentary.

If your ability to do physical work declines more than what is usual with aging, you will have more difficulty recovering from an accident or surgery should either occur. You could reach a point where activities such as standing up from a low chair or climbing stairs would require almost all your strength. You could become so weak that you can't get out of a chair or walk without help. If you lose your ability to do physical work and take care of yourself, you could lose your independence.

Keeping your heart, lungs, and muscles strong and healthy as you get older is important to your quality of health and life. People with low levels of strength and stamina have the most to gain from increasing their physical activity. A modest program of walking, cycling, or other activity that raises your heart rate will quickly improve physical fitness. Strength-building activities and activities to promote flexibility, balance, and coordination are also important parts of a balanced fitness program. A balanced fitness program is exactly what this book is about.

Do You Know?

Muscle loss begins in the mid-30s. If you are not involved in strength-building activities, you could lose about 30 percent of your original muscle tissue by the time you are 65.

Blood Vessels and Blood Pressure

Your blood vessels are similar to a rubber garden hose with water flowing through it. As the flow of water increases at the faucet, the walls of the

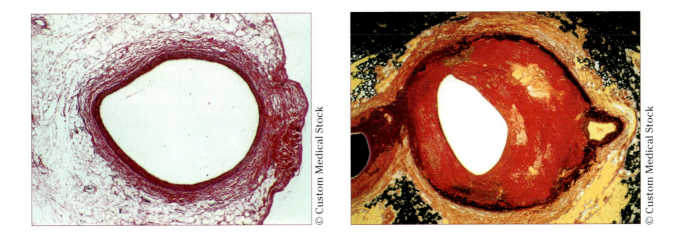

© Custom Medical Stock

© Custom Medical Stock

Compared with the healthy artery (left photo), the artery on the right is narrower and stiffer because of the disease atherosclerosis. The white area represents the clear, unobstructed part of the artery.

hose expand. As the walls of the hose expand, more water is able to flow through without unduly increasing the pressure on the hose. If something happens to cause the walls of the hose to become stiff or narrower, more resistance to the flow of water develops. The pressure inside the hose increases.

As you get older, the walls of your blood vessels become somewhat stiffer. Other changes occur in the vessels that regulate the flow of blood. Deposits of fat and cholesterol can also make the vessels narrower and reduce blood flow. This development occurs because of the disease atherosclerosis (also called hardening of the arteries) and is not due to aging. All these changes in the blood vessels cause blood pressure to rise. Fortunately, regular physical activity helps keep the blood vessels from becoming too stiff and helps maintain a normal blood pressure.

In most people, blood pressure rises with age. However, high blood pressure is not normal and should be treated. People who are physically active have lower blood pressure levels, and a physically active lifestyle helps keep blood pressure under control, even if medication is needed.

If your blood pressure is normal now, you can keep it that way by being active, maintaining a healthy weight, and eating foods low in sodium. If your blood pressure is above normal, you may be able to lower it with physical activity. Along with weight loss, physical activity is usually the first thing the doctor orders. You may even be able to lower your blood pressure enough to avoid taking medicine, or, if you need to take medicine, you may be able to take a lower dose. It is always better to control chronic health problems such as high blood pressure with lifestyle changes rather than with medication, because you'll have fewer side effects.

Do You Know?

Have you ever wondered exactly what those blood pressure numbers indicate? Here's a quick look at what they mean:

- Systolic blood pressure (the top or high number) tells the pressure of the blood against the artery walls when the heart muscle contracts to pump blood into the arteries.

- Diastolic blood pressure (the bottom or low number) tells the pressure of the blood against the artery walls when the heart is at rest (between beats).

  Normal blood pressure—systolic: less than 120, diastolic: less than 80

  Pre-high blood pressure—systolic: 120 to 139, diastolic: 80 to 89

  High blood pressure—systolic: 140 or higher, diastolic: 90 or higher

Both numbers are important. A normal resting blood pressure means that the heart is applying the proper amount of force to push the blood into the arteries and that the artery walls are not too stiff. Pre-high blood pressure means that you are likely to develop high blood pressure in the future if you don't make some changes. Take action—increase your physical activity, lose weight, eat less salt, and eat more fruit and vegetables—to reduce your blood pressure before it becomes too high.

Body Composition

Body composition describes the amounts of fat, muscle, and bone in the body. Between the ages of 30 and 70, the amount of muscle that you have decreases and the amount of fat increases. This change occurs even if your weight stays the same.

Change in body composition is important because it affects your metabolism. Metabolism is the rate at which your body burns energy (calories or kilojoules) from food. Having less muscle means that your body needs fewer calories or kilojoules to stay at the same weight.

Although some change in body composition is a common part of aging, much of the change is due to an inactive lifestyle. The extra weight can cause serious health problems. As you age, if you continue to eat the same amount of food but become less active, you will gain weight. Being overweight can cause or worsen high cholesterol, high blood pressure, and type 2 diabetes. Extra weight also causes wear and tear on the joints, particularly the knees, hips, and lower back. Regular physical activity helps protect against these problems even if you are overweight or obese. Staying active helps you maintain muscle, burn energy, and avoid gaining weight.

Bones and Joints

Problems with bones and joints are common with age. Joint and bone problems are usually linked to two conditions: osteoporosis (weak bones and fractures) and osteoarthritis (joint pain and stiffness).

If You Have Osteoporosis

If osteoporosis is untreated, bones can become so thin that they break with even mild stress. In the United States, an estimated 1.5 million fractures a year result from osteoporosis. The most common sites for fractures are the hips, lower legs and feet, wrists, and vertebrae (bones of the spine). Tiny hairline breaks in the spine can cause severe pain. Sometimes more than one vertebra is affected. Multiple fractures can reduce height by as much as 15 to 20 percent. A hump can develop in the upper portion of the spinal column, bringing the head and shoulders forward. This condition, called dowager's hump, affects 40 percent of women who have osteoporosis.

The rate of bone loss can be slowed by regular physical activity, especially strength-building activities. Eating foods rich in calcium, taking calcium supplements with vitamin D, and in women after menopause, the use of medications called bisphosponates can help prevent osteoporosis. Check your risk factors for osteoporosis in action box 3.2.

Eating foods rich in calcium is important for keeping your bones strong. Try to include at least two servings of calcium-rich foods each day. Dairy foods are excellent sources of calcium. But dairy foods made from whole milk are high in saturated fat. When selecting dairy foods, choose low-fat or nonfat sources as often as possible. Some people have difficulty digesting dairy foods because of the lactose (milk sugar) that they contain. If you can't digest lactose, drink lactose-free milk or use artificial lactase products in tablet or liquid form.

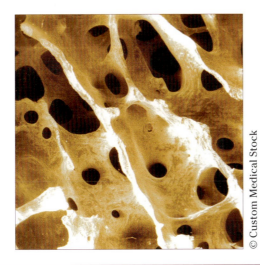
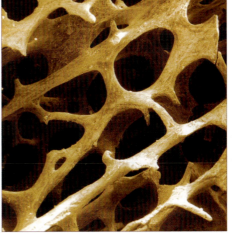

© Custom Medical Stock

Normal bone (left) and weak bone because of osteoporosis (right).

Action Box 3.2: Are You at Risk for Osteoporosis?

Mark any of the risk factors that you have. If you have risk factors for osteoporosis, you may need to have a bone density test. A bone density test is a type of X-ray that measures the amount of bone you have. In the United States, Medicare pays for bone density testing.

____Female after menopause or had ovaries removed before age 45

____Male over age 80

____Male with low levels of testosterone

____Thin or small build

____Caucasian or Asian

____Family history of osteoporosis

____Ate few calcium-rich foods (less than three glasses of milk a day) before age 30

____History of anorexia nervosa or bulimia

____History of fractures (any bone)

____Prolonged use of medicines that reduce bone strength (steroids or thyroid hormones)

____Smoke cigarettes

____Drink more than two alcoholic beverages a day

____Inactive lifestyle

Foods other than dairy foods that are good sources of calcium include broccoli, spinach, and sardines or salmon with bones. Calcium is sometimes added to foods such as orange juice, ready-to-eat cereals, and tofu, so check the food label.

Calcium supplements can make up for the calcium that you don't get from food. Talk with your doctor about whether you should take a calcium supplement. After age 50, most people need 1,500 milligrams of calcium and 400 to 800 IU (international units) of vitamin D a day. (Do not take more than 2,500 milligrams a day.) Your body needs vitamin D to help absorb calcium. Take calcium or multiple vitamin and mineral supplements that include 400 IU of vitamin D each day.

If You Have Osteoarthritis

If you have pain and stiffness in your joints, you may have osteoarthritis. Little is known about the changes of joints that occur with age. However, it

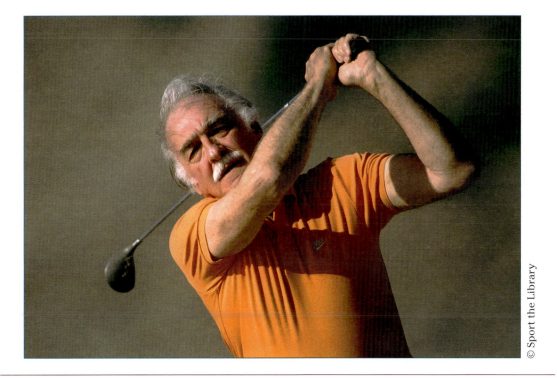

© Sport the Library

Having good flexibility allows you to move easily.

appears that most joints work well even into old age and that regular physical activity helps joints to function. Joints lose their flexibility because ligaments and tendons become less elastic. You can stay flexible with regular physical activity, especially stretching. Without good flexibility you might not be able to reach down to tie your shoes, reach up to comb your hair, or turn to back out of a parking lot.

Do You Know?

Arthritis occurs in more than 100 forms. Osteoarthritis is a disease that causes cartilage in joints to break down, leading to joint pain and stiffness. Osteoarthritis usually occurs in the hips, knees, spine, fingers, and feet. It rarely affects the wrists, elbows, shoulders, ankles, or jaw.

Osteoarthritis is common among older adults. When the cartilage is damaged by arthritis the joints become stiff and painful. People with severe pain in a joint will avoid using that joint. Although people with arthritis and other joint problems often think that physical activity and exercise are harmful, nothing could be further from the truth. Modest physical activity lessens joint pain and improves flexibility and function. Stretching, light strength training, walking, stationary cycling, swimming, and water aerobics are all excellent ways to be active without causing further joint damage or injury.

When physical activity, weight loss, and over-the-counter pain medication do not relieve pain and improve movement, ask your doctor about other therapies. These could include liniments applied to the skin, physical therapy, bracing, glucosamine and chondroitin sulfate supplements, injections of steroids, acupuncture, and in extreme cases, surgery.

Fortunately, most people can manage osteoarthritis without surgery. But for some, joint replacement is an option. A total joint replacement involves removing the arthritic or damaged joint and replacing it with an artificial joint made of plastic and metal. An X-ray or MRI is done to determine the extent of damage to the joint. An orthopedic surgeon does joint replacement surgery. Hip and knee replacements are the most common. For the knee, the damaged ends of the bones and cartilage are replaced with metal and plastic surfaces that are shaped to restore knee movement and function. For the hip, the damaged ball (the upper end of the leg bone) is replaced with a metal ball attached to a stem fitted into the leg bone. A plastic socket is implanted into the pelvis to replace the damaged socket. Joint replacements can also be performed on other joints, including the ankle, foot, shoulder, elbow, and fingers.

Personal Profile

Manuel, Age 63

Manuel has always enjoyed being active and playing sports. He played soccer in school and in recreational leagues until he was in his mid-30s. Over the years, he had several injuries to his knees. One injury required surgery. Because he now lives in a warm climate, he plays on a softball team during most of the year. You can imagine his concern when he began to experience symptoms of arthritis in his knees. He asked his primary care doctor if joint replacement surgery might be necessary. His doctor recommended a conservative approach first—physical therapy, glucosamine, and over-the-counter pain medicine. The physical therapist showed him how to do exercises to strengthen the muscles surrounding the knees. Within a few months, Manuel was moving around the bases with much less pain. Occasionally he wore a knee brace for support. Overall, he was glad that he elected a conservative approach. Understanding that softball might not always be his activity of choice, he has taken up outdoor cycling and ballroom dancing.

How to Adapt Activity for Special Conditions

If you have a health problem, you probably know it and are already under a doctor's care. Two-thirds of people 65 and older have at least one condition that requires ongoing medication or care. So, if you have a condition that must be managed, you are not alone. See table 3.1 for tips about being active if you have a special condition. You will be surprised at how easy it is to adapt a physical activity program to fit your specific needs.

Table 3.1   Being Active With Special Conditions

Health condition	Physical activity precautions and tips
High blood pressure • Causes: hardening of the arteries (atherosclerosis) and changes in the blood vessels. • Symptoms: called the silent killer because it usually has no symptoms.	• Do not exercise if your blood pressure is greater than 160/100 mmHg. See your doctor to bring it under control before increasing your activity if your blood pressure exceeds these levels. However, physical activity may be helpful in bringing your blood pressure under good control (less than 140/80) and should be part of your blood pressure control program.
	• If you take beta-blockers, you may tire easily during activity. If you do, ask your doctor if you can take a lower dose or change to a different medication to lower your blood pressure. • When doing strength-building activities, don't lift heavy weights. Use light weights and repeat the lifts more times. Be sure to breathe throughout the exercise.
Coronary heart disease • Cause: not enough blood in heart muscle because of blockages in the coronary arteries (hardening of the arteries). • Symptoms: heart pain (angina) or heart attack with physical activity.	• If you have had a heart attack or heart surgery, you should participate in a supervised cardiac rehabilitation program for the first 12 weeks after the event. Continue your activity at home or in your community after finishing cardiac rehab. • Try to avoid being physically active in places that are hot and humid. • Avoid strenuous activity at high altitudes.
Peripheral vascular disease • Cause: blockages of the arteries that carry blood to the legs. • Symptoms: pain in the calves, thigh, or buttocks during activity (called claudication). The pain usually stops when the activity is stopped. Have an exam to confirm the diagnosis. The symptoms can be confused with arthritis or nerve damage to the legs.	• Enroll in a cardiac rehabilitation program to help you get started with physical activity. People with peripheral vascular disease may also have coronary heart disease and need to be instructed in a safe program for 12 weeks. • Choose walking or stationary cycling for physical activity. These activities will lessen the pain and lengthen the time that you can be active without pain.

(continued)

Table 3.1 *Continued*

Health condition	Physical activity precautions and tips
Valvular heart disease • Cause: blocked or leaking heart valves. • Symptoms: inadequate blood supply to the rest of the body. Physical activity can cause fainting.	• Consult with a heart specialist about your physical activity.
Congestive heart failure • Cause: abnormal pumping of the heart often as a result of a heart attack. • Symptoms: backup of fluids into the lungs and other parts of the body; shortness of breath, irregular heart rhythms, and weak muscles.	• If you want to be physically active, you must do so under the supervision of a cardiac rehabilitation program.
Asthma • Cause: inflamed and narrowed bronchial tubes. • Symptoms: wheezing and shortness of breath. Physical activity may trigger asthma attacks in people with allergies (called exercise-induced asthma).	• Nearly all people with asthma can be physically active safely. • Avoid activity in severely cold, dry weather. Do physical activity in warm and more humid conditions. • In cold weather, use a face mask or scarf and breathe slowly through your nose. • If possible, don't do activity when air pollution or pollen counts are high. • Take medications if necessary. These medications are typically inhaled 15 to 30 minutes before physical activity.
Chronic obstructive pulmonary disease (COPD) • Cause: inflamed or destroyed lung tissue most often caused by years of cigarette smoking. • Symptoms: shortness of breath, chronic coughing, and frequent respiratory infections, especially during cold weather.	• Enroll in a supervised pulmonary rehabilitation program.

Health condition	Physical activity precautions and tips
Osteoarthritis • Cause: damage to the cartilage and joints of the spine, hips, knees, feet, and small joints of the hands. • Symptoms: pain and stiffness, especially when using the joint.	• Avoid activities that put too much stress on the joints, such as aerobic dancing, running, or competitive sports. • Include walking, swimming, water aerobics, stationary cycling, strength-building activities, and stretching. • Take acetaminophen, ibuprofen, or another mild pain medication 30 minutes before activity. • Avoid activities that cause too much pain to a specific joint. Choose another activity that uses different joints. • Consult an exercise specialist or a physical therapist if necessary.
Low back pain • Cause: strain to the back muscles and ligaments. More serious problems, such as spinal compression, fractures, spinal stenosis, or tumors, may also cause persistent low back pain.	• Do stretches every day to help correct muscle imbalances. • Do walking, swimming, water aerobics, and strength-building activities with light weights. • Avoid activities such as cycling, racket sports, golf, and jogging that may make back pain worse. • Stop exercising immediately if pain is acute. • Take mild pain medications as needed. Continue usual activities as much as possible. Bed rest for more than one day slows rather than helps healing. • Start your regular physical activity program again when your pain lessens.
Osteoporosis • Cause: thinning of the bones. • Symptoms: none, unless the bones become so thin that they break. Fractures most often occur in the spine, hip, lower leg, and wrist.	• Participate in weight-bearing activities such as walking and strength building to help slow bone loss. • Take a calcium supplement of least 1,500 milligrams per day with 400 to 800 IU of vitamin D. • Take bisphosphonates or other medications recommended by your doctor. • See a physical therapist to learn how to strengthen specific muscle groups around a fracture.

(continued)

Table 3.1   *Continued*

Health condition	Physical activity precautions and tips
Type 1 diabetes • Cause: buildup of high levels of glucose in the blood because the pancreas makes no insulin or very little insulin. People with type 1 diabetes must take insulin shots for the rest of their lives. • Symptoms: fatigue, frequent thirst and urination, blurred vision, rapid weight loss, and repeated infections. *Type 2 diabetes* • Cause: cells of the body resistant to insulin; buildup of high levels of glucose and insulin in the blood. • Symptoms: similar to those of type 1 diabetes.	• Monitor your blood glucose closely to prevent a low blood glucose attack after physical activity. • Carry a snack with you during activity. • Drink plenty of water to avoid dehydration. • Wear socks and shoes that fit properly and check your feet every day. • Wear identification that says you have diabetes • Don't do vigorous activity alone.
Cancer	• Don't be afraid to participate in regular activity and exercise. • Get advice from your doctor about when you can safely resume activity after surgery. • Fatigue may prevent regular activity during chemotherapy or radiation therapy. • People with lung cancer should start physical activity as part of a structured pulmonary rehabilitation program. • Stretching and building strength in the upper body is important for breast cancer survivors.
Obesity	• Avoid high-impact activities (such as jogging) that may put stress on joints. • Wear shoes that provide good support for arches. • Do strength-building activities for the legs to protect the knees from the extra stress of being overweight.

Try Affirmations

A positive attitude is essential if physical activity is to be an important part of your life. One way to develop a positive attitude is to use affirmations. Affirmations are positive statements that you repeat regularly. If you are just getting started with activity, affirmations will bolster your confidence that you can make positive changes. If you are already physically active, affirmations can help you stay active, especially during difficult situations.

You can say affirmations aloud or silently. Repeat them often with real commitment. Begin each affirmation with "I am," "I can," or "I will" rather than with "I am not." Schedule a time in your day, such as when brushing your teeth, to say affirmations. Some people believe that looking in the mirror while saying affirmations is helpful. Action box 3.3 presents a few affirmations for different stages of physical activity. Choose one or two that fit you at this time or write some of your own. Copy your affirmations on index cards and carry them in your purse or briefcase. Post them on the refrigerator or in other places where you will see them often. After a week or two, try new affirmations. Evaluate your experience with affirmations. Are you feeling more motivated to increase your physical activity? Additional affirmations will appear throughout the book.

Action Box 3.3:   Affirmations to Try

Select one or two affirmations to practice regularly this next week.

If you are just getting started with physical activity, say the following:	If you are already active and want to stay that way, say the following:
I can be more active than I am now.	I really enjoy being physically active.
I will have more energy if I'm active.	Nothing makes me feel younger than being active.
I will start to develop a plan to be more active.	Being an active person is important to me.
I will enjoy being more active.	I am healthier because I am active.
I will be healthier when I'm active.	I look and feel better because I am active.
I will have more confidence when I'm active.	I am in control of my lifestyle.
I will look and feel better when I'm active.	I will continue to be active for the rest of my life.
I'm looking forward to being more active.	I'd really miss it if I couldn't be active.
Add more affirmations here:	If I can be active, I can do anything! I am ready to tackle other challenges.
	Add more affirmations here:

Commit to an Active Lifestyle

Are you ready to start putting your thoughts into action and to do some real physical activity? Use section 1 of action box 3.4 to keep track of your thoughts and actions related to physical activity. Keeping track of and reviewing your thoughts about physical activity can help you become more physically active. You may be able to identify barriers to physical activity that you can address, or you may identify positive feelings about physical activity that you can use to motivate yourself. Answer the questions in section 2 of the action box about your physical activity thoughts when you have the thought or at the end of each day. This form also appears in the appendix, and you can make extra copies to track your thoughts and actions regularly.

Action Box 3.4: Keep Track of Your Thoughts and Actions

Part 1: Recording Thoughts and Actions

Use this form to record the number of times that you think about doing some physical activity. Simply place a mark in a box in the left column of the table each time you *think* about doing some physical activity. If you carried out your thoughts and did the activity you were thinking about, place a mark in the right column of the table.

Day	Times that I *thought* about physical activity	Times that I *followed through* on the thought and did the physical activity
Sunday		
Monday		
Tuesday		
Wednesday		
Thursday		
Friday		
Saturday		
	Total times that I thought about physical activity: _____	Total times that I followed through on the thought: _____

Part 2: Learning From Your Thoughts

1. What triggered my thought about physical activity?

   Example: I saw a friend being active.

   _____

   _____

2. What was the thought about physical activity?

   Example: "I see that Sally is walking outside. I could do that. Maybe we can walk together." Or "I see Sally walking outside. She looks cold."

   _____

   _____

3. If your thought was negative, what could you say to yourself so that you'd be more likely to be physically active?

   Example: "As long as I wear my good coat, I'll be perfectly warm."

   _____

   _____

4. If your thought was positive, did you respond by doing some physical activity? Why or why not? _____

   _____

From Active Living Partners.

Summary

In this chapter you learned about some of the changes that occur after age 50, both those that are expected and those that are not. Physical activity can slow or delay usual aging and prevent many of the health problems that are common as you get older. If you have a condition that must be managed, physical activity may reduce your symptoms and prevent complications. In fact, people with special conditions stand to gain the most from being physically active. Remember: You can age fast or age slow. It's up to you.

The remainder of this book will help you develop a balanced physical activity program to fit your specific needs.

Chapter Checklist

Following are some ways in which you can apply what you learned in this chapter to your daily life. Over the next few days and weeks try to do as many of these activities as possible.

- ❏ Consider how you might adapt your physical activity program if you have a special health problem.

- ❏ Write a few affirmations about physical activity and repeat them when you brush your teeth every morning and night for at least one week. They will become your inner dialogues.

- ❏ Start keeping track of your thoughts and actions about physical activity.

- ❏ Review your list of pros and cons for physical activity. Can you add at least one more pro to your list?

Word Search

See if you can find 10 important words from this chapter in the grid that follows. Words appear forward and backward in rows, columns, and diagonals. The solution is shown on page 231.

```
S  T  G  E  L  R  H  L  X  X  E  I  W  L  S
A  N  L  A  V  P  O  J  M  Q  M  H  O  I  I
F  E  O  H  G  D  S  U  F  Q  I  S  T  P  G
F  V  P  I  S  I  I  C  Z  Y  T  I  B  B  Q
I  E  V  M  T  C  N  Z  L  E  R  V  H  C  P
R  R  A  U  L  C  Q  G  O  H  G  S  J  L  O
M  P  R  A  X  V  A  P  T  O  Q  N  O  O  Z
A  K  C  J  M  U  O  R  D  E  L  A  Y  U  F
T  W  T  Q  N  R  A  O  Z  C  Y  L  N  J  S
I  J  B  L  O  O  D  P  R  E  S  S  U  R  E
O  G  A  S  E  L  M  H  E  S  T  E  G  I  U
N  X  I  T  S  T  H  G  U  O  H  T  W  L  S
S  S  S  Z  I  O  Q  E  F  Q  R  N  C  M  R
E  O  L  F  U  L  O  O  S  B  X  G  S  Z  M
R  Y  Z  U  D  W  O  E  X  X  Q  P  V  W  V
```

Actions   Calcium   Osteoporosis
Affirmations   Delay   Prevent
Aging   Osteoarthritis   Thoughts
Blood pressure

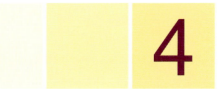

Step It Up

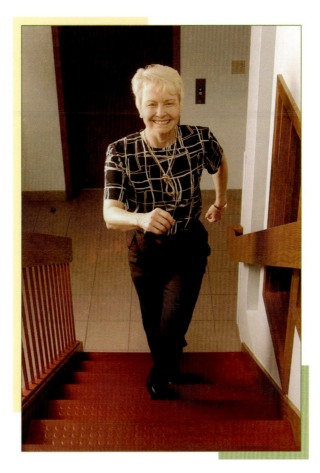

In This Chapter

❏ Use a step counter to assess your overall physical activity.

❏ Be aware of times when you are inactive and active.

❏ Learn time management skills.

❏ Find time to fit in short bouts of activity.

W e hope that you are eager to increase your physical activity. But first, take a little time to assess your current level of physical activity. Knowing your physical activity level will help you in three ways:

- Having a clear view of your current level of activity will allow you to set realistic goals for the future.

- Activity logs will help you recognize your progress over time. Seeing your success will keep you motivated.

- Monitoring your activity will itself be motivational. People who regularly keep activity logs, especially when they are getting started, are more likely to be successful with their program than people who don't keep records.

In this chapter you'll learn several ways to keep track of the amount of physical activity that you are doing. You'll also learn how to fit in short bouts of activity. Find which methods appeal to you and try them.

Research News You Can Use

Question: Does stair climbing benefit your health?

Answer: In the College Alumni Study (Paffenbarger and Lee 1998), men who climbed more than 20 flights of stairs per week had about a 10 percent lower death rate than did men who climbed fewer than 20 flights of stairs. This reduction in risk of dying was after taking into account other types and amounts of physical activity, such as walking and sports.

In Northern Ireland, young women who climbed stairs over the course of seven weeks improved their fitness and increased their HDL ("good") cholesterol levels (Boreham, Wallace, and Nevill 2000).

How you can use this news: To improve your health and reduce your risk of dying, start taking the stairs instead of the elevator or escalator. Locate the stairs in buildings that you visit often. Climb to your floor, *especially* if you are going no more than three or four flights. After you become more fit, extend the number of flights of stairs that you climb. If you are going up more than four or five floors, get off the elevator a few floors early and climb the stairs the rest of the way. You'll save time and burn extra energy.

Count Your Daily Steps

Counting the number of steps you take each day is a useful way to monitor your overall physical activity level, and doing so is easy if you use a step counter (pedometer). You can wear one of these small, lightweight devices on your belt or waistband. Step counters are available in most sporting-goods stores for about $20. You can also purchase step counters at http://aarp.stepuptobetterhealth.com/. A step counter will not accurately measure the distance that you walk, but it will record the number of steps you take—up and down, little steps and giant ones. Some step counters do not count steps reliably. Several brands have been shown to be accurate. See www.pedometers.com for an evaluation of various step counters.

First, determine your baseline, the average number of steps you take each day. Wear your step counter for one week while following your normal routine. Record the number of steps per day on the chart in action box 4.1. At the end of the week, find the average number of steps per day to establish your baseline. Your goal is to find ways to increase this number by building more activity into your daily routine. Continue to record your steps each day as you increase your physical activity.

Do You Know?

The average number of steps that inactive people take per day is usually in the range of 2,500 to 5,000. An unusually inactive day will result in only 1,500 to 2,000 steps. If the day involves more moving around than normal, perhaps when traveling and walking in airports, the number of steps will likely be higher.

If your daily routine has not included much activity and you can work up to a total of 8,000 to 12,000 steps per day on average, you will be getting enough physical activity to obtain important health benefits.

Follow these tips for using a step counter:

- Keep the case closed while wearing the step counter. Open it only to check your readings. Most step counters will not count steps if the case is open.

- Avoid dropping the step counter or getting it wet. Some people like to attach a string or ribbon to the step counter so that they can pin it to their clothing.

- If you attach your step counter to your underwear, be careful when using the toilet. You may have to go fishing!

- Do a test to be sure that the step counter is counting steps properly. Attach the step counter. Walk 50 steps. Check the number of steps recorded. If it is not off by more than three steps either way (47 to 53), that's good enough. If the number of steps is not within this range, move

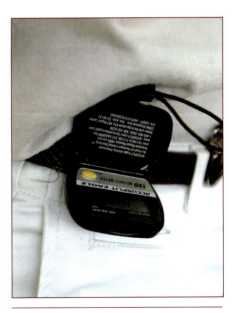

Attach a step counter to your belt or waistband in a horizontal position above the middle of your thigh. Keep it closed while you walk.

the step counter to another position and try again. The step counter is not likely to count accurately if you

- shuffle your feet,
- ride a bicycle, or
- bounce up and down.

Action Box 4.1: How Many Steps Do You Take Each Day?

Use this form to record your steps each day for one week. Compare your activity on weekdays and weekends. At the end of the week, find your average steps per day by dividing your total number of steps by seven. That figure is your baseline. How can you increase the number of steps that you take each day? Write your ideas in the space provided. Set a goal for increasing your daily steps.

	Sun.	Mon.	Tue.	Wed.	Thu.	Fri.	Sat.	Average
Steps per day								
(Example)	3,578	1,094	1,372	1,255	1,106	1,289	4,122	1,974

Ways in which I will increase my steps each day:

_____

_____

_____

My goal for next week is an average of _____ steps per day.

_____

Do You Know?

Waiting for and riding in an elevator burns about 1.5 calories (6 kilojoules) per minute for a 175-pound (79-kilogram) person. The same person could use 8 or 9 calories per minute (34 to 38 kilojoules per minute) climbing stairs. Over time, this small change could make a big difference.

Find Time to Be Active

When asked why they aren't more active, many people say that they don't have enough time. Indeed, life is busy. Demands on your time are considerable. But everyone has the same amount of time—60 minutes an hour, 24 hours a day, and 168 hours per week. The choices that you make about how you spend your time say a lot about your values and priorities. The average adult in the United States watches more than five hours of TV each day. That's a lot of time spent sitting. Obviously, time is available for other pursuits. Couldn't people use 30 minutes for physical activity? The issue is a matter of priorities. Even many world leaders, extremely busy people indeed, recognize the importance of being active and make time for regular physical activity. If they can find time, so can you!

Do a Personal Time Study

The personal time study in action box 4.2 will help you become more aware of how you spend your time (active versus inactive). Carry out studies for two typical weekdays and one typical weekend day. You will use the results of these time studies later in this chapter. Examples are given for Ben and Candice. They used their personal time studies to find ways to be more active.

Later you may want to repeat the studies, so make extra copies of the form for future use. A blank form is provided in the appendix.

Action Box 4.2: Personal Time Study

Make three copies of the time form. Fill in the time slots with the tasks or activities that you do over three typical days (two weekdays and one weekend day). After you've recorded your activities, determine the number of minutes that you spent doing any type of physical activity—walking, climbing stairs, gardening, housework—and your minutes of inactivity, such as sleeping, sitting, riding in a car or bus, watching television, or talking on the phone. At the bottom on the form, add up the minutes of activity (Yes column) and inactivity (No column) for the day. The total for each four-hour time slot should be 240 minutes. The total for each day should be 1,440 minutes.

		PHYSICALLY ACTIVE?	
Time slot	Tasks or activities	Yes	No
Midnight to 4:00 a.m.			
4:00 to 8:00 a.m.			
8:00 a.m. to noon			
Noon to 4:00 p.m.			
4:00 to 8:00 p.m.			
8:00 p.m. to midnight			
		Total minutes of activity:	Total minutes of inactivity:

(continued)

➡**Action Box 4.2: Personal Time Study** *(continued)*

Instead of (inactive times)   I will do (list activities here)

■ _____   ■ _____

■ _____   ■ _____

■ _____   ■ _____

Reprinted from S. Blair, A. Dunn, B. Marcus, R.A. Carpenter, and P. Jaret, 2001, *Active living every day* (Champaign, IL: Human Kinetics), 184.

Personal Profiles

Ben, Age 59

Ben works for an insurance company. He works a typical 40-hour workweek. His personal time studies (examples #1 and #2) show his minutes of activity on a typical weekday before and after making changes in his lifestyle. Only two segments of his time study are shown.

EXAMPLE #1, BEN (BEFORE)		PHYSICALLY ACTIVE?	
Time slot	Tasks or activities	Yes	No
Noon to 4:00 p.m.	Eat lunch, visit with coworkers.		50
	Walk back to office.	5	
	Call coworkers to check progress on projects.		45
	Work at desk, writing reports and talking on phone.		140
4:00 to 8:00 p.m.	Conduct meeting in my office with coworkers.		60
	Walk from office to elevator for parking garage.	5	
	Drive home.		45
	Change into casual clothes and read the newspaper.		40
	Help prepare dinner, eat dinner, and clean kitchen.		50
	Watch TV with spouse.		40
	Totals for segments shown (minutes):	10	470

Instead of (inactive times)   I will do (list activities here)

Visiting at lunch   Invite coworkers to go for a walk and visit

Meeting   Walk while problem solving

Reading the newspaper   Walk and talk with spouse

	EXAMPLE #2, BEN (AFTER)	PHYSICALLY ACTIVE?	
Time slot	Tasks or activities	Yes	No
Noon to 4:00 p.m.	Eat lunch with coworkers.		30
	Invite coworkers to go for a walk together after lunch.	20	
	Walk back to office.	5	
	Walk to other offices to check progress on projects.	10	35
	Work at desk, writing reports and talking on phone (stretch while talking).	5	135
4:00 to 8:00 p.m.	Conduct meeting in office with coworkers.		60
	Walk from office to parking garage, take stairs.	5	
	Drive home.		45
	Change into casual clothes, go for a walk with spouse while talking.	30	10
	Help prepare dinner, eat dinner, and clean kitchen.		50
	Listen to music and discuss vacation plans with spouse.		40
	Totals for segments shown (minutes):	**75**	**405**

Candice, Age 61

Candice and her husband are retired. One morning a week, she looks after her four-year-old grandson while his mom does errands. Her personal time studies (examples #3 and #4) show how she added 30 minutes of physical activity in a block of time during which she was previously inactive. As a bonus, her grandson enjoyed some physical activity too!

	EXAMPLE #3, CANDICE (BEFORE)	PHYSICALLY ACTIVE?	
Time slot	Tasks or activities	Yes	No
8:00 a.m. to noon	Daughter drops off grandson (four years old) for the morning.		
	Watch cartoons with grandson.		45
	Play board games or cards.		30
	Prepare snack and eat it together.	5	25
	Write letters and e-mails while grandson plays alone or watches TV.		60
	Have coffee and visit with daughter for a while before she leaves to return home.		45
	Make phone calls to friends.		30
	Total for the segment shown (minutes):	**5**	**235**

(continued)

Instead of (inactive times)   I will (list activities here)

Play board games   Walk with my grandson to the park and push him on the swing

EXAMPLE #4, CANDICE (AFTER)		PHYSICALLY ACTIVE?	
Time slot	Tasks or activities	Yes	No
8:00 a.m. to noon	Daughter drops off grandson (four years old) for the morning.		
	Watch cartoons with grandson.		45
	Walk with grandson to a park in the neighborhood. Push him on the swing. Play other active games.	20	
	Return home, walking while encouraging grandson to skip some of the way.	10	
	Prepare a snack and eat it together.	5	25
	Give grandson a bath and read a story.	5	25
	Write letters, e-mails, or make phone calls to friends while grandson plays alone.		60
	Have coffee and visit with daughter for a while before she leaves to return home.		45
	Total for the segment shown (minutes):	40	200

What did you learn from your personal time study about how you use your time? Chances are that the amount of time you spend being physically inactive surprised you. If you want to fit more physical activity into your day but are not sure how to do it, keep reading!

Review Your Commitments

Do time pressures make you feel stressed and anxious? For busy people, time management is an effective way to reduce stress and find ways to fit in physical activity. Use the three personal time studies that you have already completed as you work through action box 4.3. You can review your commitments and then think about any adjustments that you may want to make.

Action Box 4.3: Consider Your Commitments

Use your records from your three personal time studies to identify your major commitments. Calculate the amount of time you spent in each of the three major life areas. The total for the three areas should equal 72 hours for the three days.

Productive and work time—includes time on the job, volunteer work, commuting to and from work, job-related work at home, errands, working around the house (cleaning, cooking, and so on), and other work or productive tasks

Time with others and relationships—includes time interacting with others (spouse, children, parents, other friends or family members), time spent in parenting or caretaking activities, and any other nonwork social activity

Personal time—includes time sleeping, napping, relaxing, grooming and practicing personal hygiene, being physically active, reading for pleasure, meditating, worshiping, and doing other things for yourself

EXAMPLE #1 FOR BEN			
Day	**Productive or work time**	**Time with others or relationships**	**Personal time**
Weekday	9 hours 45 minutes	1 hour 50 minutes	12 hours 25 minutes

Day	**Productive or work time**	**Time with others or relationships**	**Personal time**
Weekday	_____ hours	_____ hours	_____ hours
Weekday	_____ hours	_____ hours	_____ hours
Weekend day	_____ hours	_____ hours	_____ hours
Total hours = 72	_____ hours	_____ hours	_____ hours

See Ben's personal time study (example #1, p. 58) before he increased his activity. Ben realized that he didn't spend much quality time with his spouse on workdays. As shown in example #2, he suggested that they take a walk together after work and visit about the events of the day. They also decided to turn off the television after dinner and listen to music while discussing plans for an active vacation.

Check Your Balance

Balance is a term frequently used in discussions of time management. Are you dividing your time and energy fairly (not necessarily evenly) among the three important life areas—productivity and work, relationships, and personal? Some people become compulsive about work and other productive endeavors. They go beyond enjoying and being committed to their work. Do you have any of these characteristics? Do you

- feel guilty if you are not engaged in productive work,
- have difficulty enjoying free or unstructured time,
- blame someone else for why you must work so much, or
- deny that you have any control over your workload?

Relationships with others are critical to your well-being. But, like work and productivity, too much of a good thing can lead to imbalance. Some people spend a lot of time and energy doing for others. They neglect themselves and their work. Do you have any of these characteristics? Do you

- feel that you must anticipate and meet the needs of everyone around you,
- allow others to be overly dependent on you, or
- feel that the more you do, the more others expect from you?

Taking care of yourself is the foundation for productivity and rewarding relationships. All areas are interrelated. Do you have any of these characteristics? Do you

- feel guilty if you take time for yourself,
- hold others responsible for your personal needs,
- neglect your grooming and personal hygiene, or
- use food, alcohol, or tobacco to relieve stress?

Finding time for regular physical activity is part of taking care of yourself. When you take time to care for yourself, you'll probably be surprised at how much more you accomplish all around. Do you currently overemphasize or underemphasize an aspect of your life? In either case, identify one change that you can make this week to bring your commitments more in line with the balance that you'd like to have. Write what you will do in action box 4.4.

Action Box 4.4: What I Will Do to Achieve Balance in My Life

Example for Ben:

This week, I will take the following actions to achieve balance in my life:

- *Go for a walk with my wife after work and talk about the day's events*
- *Turn off the TV after dinner and spend time talking with my wife*
- *Start to make plans for an active vacation together*

This week, I will take the following actions to achieve balance in my life:

- _____

  _____

- _____

  _____

- _____

  _____

Use Time More Efficiently

No matter how many demands or responsibilities you have, you can find ways to use your time more efficiently. Practicing good time management will improve your physical and mental health. You'll feel in control of your life and be able to find the time to be active without compromising your other responsibilities or interests. See the time management tips in the following list. Select one or two of the tips to try during the next week.

Time Management Tips

- Set priorities. Organize tasks by what you must do, what you hope to do, and what you will do if you have the time.

- Don't overcommit. Learn to protect your time by setting limits. Say no without feeling guilty.

- Try to give up on some of your perfectionist ways. Acceptable outcomes can take less time.

- Spend some time getting organized. Could you develop a system for paying your bills? Would a better organized closet help when you must pack for a business trip or vacation?

- Arrange your work time efficiently. Do difficult tasks when your energy is at its peak. Always do major tasks first. Match the task to the time available.

- Learn to negotiate and delegate jobs to others. Ask for help if you need it. Chapter 8 provides more about getting support from others.

(continued)

Fit in Lifestyle Physical Activity

You can fit in bouts of physical activity of 5 to 15 minutes in hundreds of ways. Most come under the umbrella of lifestyle physical activity rather than structured exercise, but such activities count too. Look back at your personal time studies. Complete action box 4.5 to plan ways in which you can fit in extra bouts of physical activity throughout your day. Recall how Ben and Candice were able to fit in a lot more activity during the day without compromising their work or personal responsibilities. Here are a few ideas. Do any of them appeal to you?

At Home

- Do common household chores with extra vigor. Really push and pull the vacuum or do lunges. Think of chores as workouts.

- Plan inefficiencies. Make extra trips when unloading the groceries, taking out the garbage, or picking up and putting away.

- Take a walk around the block before getting the mail from the mailbox.

- Walk or cycle, instead of drive, to do errands for one item. Walking or cycling may at times be easier than looking for a parking place.

- Volunteer for projects in your neighborhood—creating a walking trail, planting trees, picking up litter, or building playground structures.

At Work

- Plan to arrive a few minutes early so that you can park farther from the entrance.

- Ride the bus but get off a few blocks early and walk the rest of the way.

- Organize a walking group among coworkers.

- Set a timer on your computer or watch to remind you to get up and move frequently.

- Deliver a message in person rather than calling.

- Manage projects or supervise others by walking around.

- Walk or do stretches while talking on the phone. Use resistance rubber bands to do a few strength-building exercises. Books can serve as hand weights.

- Stay a little later at the end of the day. Take a short walk before heading home. You may avoid the worst traffic.

During Travel and Leisure

- Walk through the airport terminal while waiting for your flight.

- Select hotels that have a pool or fitness room and plan time in your schedule to use the facilities.

- Plan walking sightseeing trips—to museums and botanical gardens, through historical areas, along nature trails.

- Play games with young children that get both of you active. For example, a scavenger hunt is a fun way to walk.

- At spectator sports, walk along the sidelines rather than sit in the bleachers.

- Get involved in an active hobby, such as golf, gardening, woodworking, dancing, or canoeing.

- Serve as an usher at theater, concert, or sporting events.

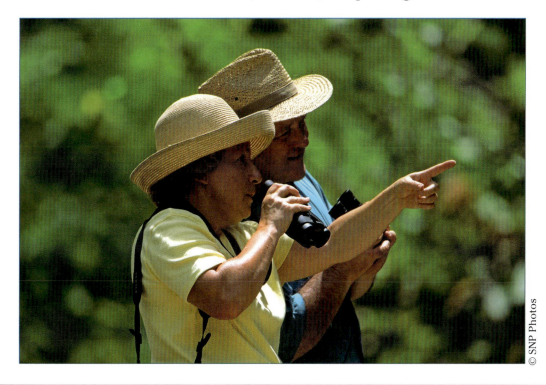

© SNP Photos

When traveling, plan walking sightseeing trips, like this one along a nature trail.

Action Box 4.5: My Ways to Fit In Fitness

List a total of five new ways in which you will incorporate lifestyle physical activity into your daily routine. Be specific. For example, rather than saying that you will walk after work, say, "I will walk around the block at least once before starting to read the newspaper." Try to do activities that are the same intensity as brisk walking. Aim for at least five minutes of additional physical activity at a time.

Ways that I will be active at home:

1. _____

_____

2. _____

_____

3. _____

_____

Ways that I will be active at work:

1. _____

_____

2. _____

_____

3. _____

_____

Ways that I will be active through recreation and leisure:

1. _____

_____

2. _____

_____

3. _____

_____

Summary

In this chapter, we introduced the step counter as a tool to help you assess your current physical activity level and monitor how you spend your time. Were you surprised by how much time you spend in inactive pursuits? Wearing a step counter can help you become more aware of your overall activity and find ways to take extra steps. If you are like most people, practicing time management is key to increasing your physical activity. Practicing time management also reduces stress and gives you a sense of balance and control in your life.

The next chapter focuses on specific ways in which you can get organized for physical activity. You will need to select the right shoes and clothing. You will also learn how to arrange your home and surroundings to be more supportive of your new habit. You can remind yourself to be active.

Chapter Checklist

Following are some ways in which you can apply what you have learned in this chapter to your daily life. Over the next few days and weeks try to do as many of these activities as possible.

❑ Assess how much time you are inactive. Start to think of ways you can substitute activity for inactivity. Use the form from chapter 3, Keeping Track of Your Thoughts, to record your thoughts about physical activity as well as your actions.

❑ Get a step counter and use it to count your daily steps over a period of a week. Set a goal to increase your daily steps. Continue to wear the step counter and monitor your steps. Write your daily steps on your personal calendar.

❑ Evaluate how you spend your time by completing the personal time study. Make adjustments that will allow time for activity. Use some of the time management tips.

❑ Think of at least five new ways to fit in more lifestyle physical activity at home, at work, and during leisure time and then put them into action.

Word Search

See if you can find 10 important words from this chapter in the grid that follows. Words appear forward and backward in rows, columns, and diagonals. The solution is shown on page 231.

```
W T P N H J M U Y H G C I L B
C L I M B I N G S T A I R S R
G S Z M G A K N Y J S E Y T I
U S T W E Y L Y D E X S Z U S
J J I N Y M F A I Y T H H O K
X Z N K E D A T N E R K C B W
M B M L S M I N P C T Q O T A
Z G F T P R T C A X E Z L R L
S H A A O M O I V G Y Y R O K
M P L I B U Y Q M B E J A H I
R N R N N A L E Z M T M J S N
G P G T N K Q B L V O V E F G
D D E L E G A T E U D C B N K
O R Y A W A R A F K R A P D T
H L O H R Z C C E E X B L B K
```

Balance	Delegate	Short bouts
Brisk walking	Park far away	Step counter
Climbing stairs	Priorities	Time management
Commitments		

Organize Yourself

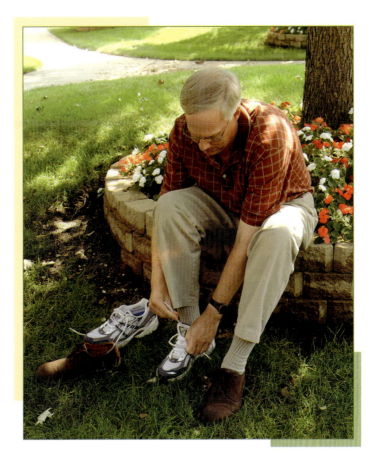

In This Chapter

- ❑ Select shoes and clothing for activity.
- ❑ Organize your home and surroundings to promote activity.
- ❑ Remind yourself to be active every day.
- ❑ Think about rewards that would motivate you to be more active.
- ❑ Set a short-term goal to increase your physical activity.

Now that you've considered how you can fit more activity into your lifestyle, you'll want to be ready when an opportunity presents itself. The most essential thing you need to be active is comfortable shoes and the right clothes. But you don't have to wait for opportunities to present themselves to be active. You can take actions to remind yourself to be active. People who are active on most days of the week have organized their surroundings to promote and support their habits.

Shoes for Activity

You should always wear comfortable, supportive shoes. You aren't going to change into athletic shoes for climbing the stairs, nor are you likely to walk, instead of drive, to do a quick errand if walking is going to make your feet hurt. Ideally, you should be able to wear comfortable shoes all day, every day.

Many shoe companies make attractive dress shoes that have the support and cushioning necessary for walking for extended periods. Choose dress shoes that you can walk in for 10 minutes or even two hours. When you find a style that you like, buy several pairs, perhaps in different colors. Women should select shoes with the lowest heel possible. Men should choose a lace-up style rather than a loafer so that they can adjust the tightness and maximize support. See the tips for selecting the right shoes on the next page.

Besides buying comfortable shoes for every day, you may want to buy athletic shoes for occasions when you plan to do extended bouts of activity. Some athletic shoes, typically called cross-training shoes, are designed for a variety of activities. Other shoes are designed for specific activities to meet demands such as the following:

- Impact—The shoe should provide adequate cushioning for the foot when it hits the ground.

- Vertical or lateral motion—The shoe should meet the particular demands of the activity, such as the repetitive vertical movement of walking or jogging or the side-to-side movement of tennis or basketball.

- Risk of ankle sprain—For some activities, the shoe should provide extra protection against the risk of twisting an ankle.

To illustrate the differences among various types of shoes, let's compare shoes for walking, tennis, and group fitness classes.

- Walking shoes can be of almost any style. They need only mild heel elevation, good support in the arch, a snug heel, and a roomy toe box. The width of a thumb between the largest toe and the end of the shoe will ensure sufficient length. A beveled heel can make for a smooth heel strike with good flexibility in the forefoot for an easier push off the toe.

- Tennis shoes need adequate cushioning in the midsole to absorb the shock in both the heel and forefoot. A durable outside is needed to resist the wear from starting and stopping. A special toe cap can limit abrasion from the toe drag that occurs during the serve. Most important, tennis shoes also need a broad base of support for side-to-side movements and extra ankle support.

■ Shoes for group fitness classes need plenty of cushioning in the midsole, especially in the forefoot where the impact is concentrated. Good flexibility and a broad base of support are also important. For step classes, a shoe with a slightly higher top offers greater lateral support and helps reduce the risk of ankle sprains.

Tips for Selecting the Right Shoes

■ If you are selecting athletic shoes for the first time, shop at a store that has sales people who can give personal service rather than at a self-help, discount store. The sales person should be able to answer your questions and fit you into a shoe best suited to your needs.

■ Shop at a store that has a variety of brands and types of shoes.

■ Try on shoes at the end of the day when your feet are likely to be larger.

■ Take along the type of sock that you'll be wearing with the shoes.

■ Select a shoe with a removable insole if you'll be wearing orthotic devices.

■ Spread and wiggle your toes to be sure that you have ample room in the toe box. Your longest toe should be about the width of a thumb from the end of the shoe.

■ Lace your shoes and check the space between the lace holes across the tongue of the shoe. About one inch (2.54 centimeters) of space between the lace holes provides the appropriate fit. Less space means that the shoes are too big, and you don't have room to tighten the shoe. More than an inch may mean that the shoes are too narrow or tight.

■ Stand on your tiptoes to be sure that the heels don't slip.

■ Check the arch of the shoe. The arch should support the arch of your foot.

■ Walk or jog around the store to test for comfort and cushioning, preferably on a hard surface instead of carpet.

■ Take the shoes home and wear them for a few hours, preferably late in the day. Try them out during your activity of choice. If they don't feel good, take them back to the store and get fitted again.

If you find a shoe that works well for you, stay with that model. Buy an extra pair for future use or to alternate with your first pair. If your feet perspire heavily, alternate pairs to allow one pair to air and dry thoroughly. Two pairs of shoes worn on alternate days will last more than twice as long as one pair of shoes worn every day.

Check Your Shoes and Feet

How your shoes wear tells a lot about your feet and the kind of shoes you need. Place your shoes side by side on a flat surface. How do your shoes wear? Most shoes will show some wear on the outside of the heel, but note these distinctions:

- Normal–shoes sit relatively straight and wear evenly.
- Overpronate–shoes tilt to the inside and show wear under the big toe and on the inside edge of the forefoot.
- Underpronate–shoes tilt to the outside and show wear along the outsides from the toes to the heels.

Table 5.1 shows an easy way to know whether you require shoes with special features.

If you have ever heard avid runners talk about their running shoes, you'd think they were talking about tires for their cars. Runners know how many miles they can expect to get from a pair of shoes. All athletic shoes will last for only a limited time. You need new shoes when

- the tread pattern is worn,
- the lateral heel wears through to the foam midsole,
- the toe box is thin or worn,
- your feet feel tired after activity, especially in the arches,

Table 5.1 How Do Your Shoes Wear?

Alignment	Condition	Solution
Normal	Your forefoot and heel are perfectly aligned with the ground and lower leg when in motion.	No specific stability or motion-control features are necessary.
Overpronate	Your foot leans excessively inward. The outer side of your foot hits the ground first and rolls inward with each stride.	You need shoes that provide extra stability and motion-control features.
Underpronate	Your foot leans excessively outward. The outer side of your foot hits the ground first and continues to roll outward to push off.	You need lots of cushioning because your foot does not pronate (roll inward) enough to absorb impact properly. You also need durable cushioning because the impact forces are mainly on the sides of your feet.

- you feel pain in the shins, knees, and hips after activity, or
- you have worn the shoes regularly for 10 to 12 months or have walked 500 miles.

Personal Profile

Gerry, Age 75

Gerry has run 21 marathons, but now he mostly walks with occasional jogging. If you were to meet Gerry, you would know right away that he has an active lifestyle. He looks slim and fit and has a bounce in his step. Even when dressed in a sports jacket and tie, he wears athletic shoes. It's his trademark. At any time, Gerry probably owns three or four pairs of athletic shoes. He keeps them wherever he is likely to be active—at the lake cabin, in the boat, in his pickup truck, in the garage, in his wife's car, in a workout bag. He is never without the right shoes for physical activity.

Take Care of Your Feet

Years of wear and tear, as well as shoes that don't fit properly, are the most common causes of foot problems in older adults. Rheumatoid arthritis or osteoarthritis, poor circulation in the feet, deformities, and gout (another type of arthritis) can cause other problems. See table 5.2 for information about some common foot problems and their causes and symptoms. Tips for prevention and treatment of these specific problems are also provided. Your feet don't have to hurt or keep you from being active.

To keep your feet healthy, follow these additional tips:

- Wash your feet with warm water (not hot) and mild soap. Dry your feet with a soft towel (between the toes too!).
- Use a cream to massage and moisturize your feet.
- Put antifungus powder between your toes to keep them dry and clean.
- File toenails straight across with a slight curve at the corners.
- See your doctor or a podiatrist (foot specialist) for removal of corns or calluses.
- Choose shoes with the upper parts made of soft, flexible material to match the shape of your foot. Shoes with nonslippery soles and low heels are comfortable and safe.
- Break in new shoes slowly.
- Walk around some every hour to improve circulation (and burn a few extra calories!).

Table 5.2 Common Foot Problems Among Older Adults

Condition	Cause or symptoms	Prevention or treatment
Fungal and bacterial conditions, including athlete's foot	Causes redness, blisters, peeling, and itching. If not treated properly, an infection may get worse and be difficult to cure.	Keep your feet clean and dry, especially the area between the toes. Expose your feet to air. Dust your feet daily with a fungicidal powder. For severe or recurring cases, see your doctor for a prescription antifungal medication.
Corns and calluses	Caused by the friction and pressure of bony areas rubbing against shoes.	Wear shoes that fit properly. Use special pads. Do not attempt to treat these conditions yourself, especially if you have diabetes or poor circulation.
Bunions	Develop when the big toe joints are out of line and become swollen and tender.	Wear shoes cut wide at the instep. Use whirlpool baths. Talk with your doctor about injections or surgery.
Ingrown toenails	Caused by improperly trimmed nails.	Cut toenails straight across and level with the tip of the toes.
Yellowed toe nails	Age-related or caused by fungus.	Usually does not require treatment.
Spurs	Caused by muscle strain in the feet; irritated by standing for long periods, wearing shoes that don't fit properly, or being overweight.	Use proper foot support, heel pads, heel cups.

If you have pain in your lower leg (shins) or knees that is worse after you've been on your feet a lot, you may benefit from orthotics. Orthotics are inserts that you put in your shoes to change the position of your feet and correct foot problems. People with fallen arches (flat feet) are most likely to need orthotics. Orthotics come in many types. Some are custom made by podiatrists or physical therapists to fit your feet and shoes. Others, such as molds or arch supports, are available over the counter.

In extreme cases, surgery may be necessary to correct foot problems. Although sometimes successful, surgery is usually painful. Surgery also limits your standing and walking for weeks to months. You should consider foot surgery only after other measures have failed. If you must have foot surgery, be sure to do non-weight-bearing activities such as stationary cycling to maintain your muscle strength and stamina while your feet heal.

Diabetes, a common health problem among people over age 50, can cause serious foot problems if it is not managed. Diabetes can decrease the blood supply to the feet and reduce feeling. Cuts or sores on the feet may go unnoticed and not heal properly. In the worst cases, amputations may be necessary. If you have diabetes, you need to examine your feet carefully every day. Use a mirror to check the bottoms of your feet or ask someone else to check them for you. Look for the following:

- Changes in temperature—hot spots
- Changes in size—swelling or tenderness anywhere you apply hand pressure
- Breaks in the skin—blisters, cuts, sores, or cracks between the toes
- Color changes—blue, bright red, or white (pale) spots

Special foot care tips for people with diabetes are provided in the following list.

Special Foot Care Tips for People With Diabetes

Do the Following:

- Check the inside of your shoes each day for rough areas or foreign objects.
- Watch out for rocks, stones, curbs, and furniture legs.
- Always wear socks and change them every day.
- Throw away mended socks or socks with holes.
- Choose synthetic moisture-wicking socks with light elastic around the ankles.
- Keep your feet warm. Wear socks to bed.

Don't Do the Following:

- Cut your nails short.
- Soak or scrub your feet or put them in hot water.
- Leave hand cream or lotion between your toes.
- Use hot water bottles, heating pads, or electric blankets on your feet.
- Use adhesive tape on your feet.
- Wear socks with thick seams or turn them inside out to smooth the seams around the toes.
- Wear cotton socks. They tend to absorb sweat and be less abrasive.
- Wear high-heel or open-toed shoes or go barefoot, even at the beach.
- Use drying medicines like iodine, rubbing alcohol, Epsom salts, or peroxide on your feet.

Clothes for Activity

Where you will be physically active largely determines what you wear for physical activity. For indoor activity at home, in your neighborhood, or at the health club, choose anything that you feel comfortable wearing. Remember, an advantage of lifestyle activity—those short bouts of activity that you fit in throughout your day—is that you don't have to change clothing. You can do it in whatever you are wearing, wherever you are.

What you wear is most important for outdoor activity. For outdoor activity, remember the four Ls:

- Light-colored
- Loose-fitting
- Lightweight
- Layered

If the air is warm, dress in loose-fitting, light-colored, quick-drying fabrics. If the air is cold, dress in lightweight layers. Insulated air trapped beneath several thin layers of clothing keeps you warmer than a single thick layer does. You can add or subtract layers as needed.

Avoid wearing cotton or wool as the first layer. These fibers absorb moisture and keep it next to your skin so that you feel clammy or cold. Choose polypropylene fabric, which wicks sweat or water away from the skin or toward an outer layer of clothing. Add a layer of wool or synthetic fabric for warmth. Keep it loose for freedom and movement. An outer shell can keep wind and water out and inner layers dry. If you are likely to get wet, take special precautions, especially if the weather is cold. Rainwear should have latex rubber gaskets at neck, wrists, and ankles to prevent cold water from getting to the skin and clothing. Front zippers can be a source of leaks, so consider a pullover jacket with a hood. Remember, staying dry means staying warm and comfortable.

During outdoor activities, you may want to wear a small pack that you can strap around your waist to carry a few extra items, such as a snack, a small amount of money, keys, identification, sunscreen, and a handkerchief. If you aren't sure about places to stop for water along the way, plan to carry water. Water carriers with shoulder straps make it easy to carry water with you. Other outdoor activities and sports, such as cycling, trail hiking, canoeing, swimming, skiing, racket sports, and golf, each have a unique set of clothing and gear requirements.

Dehydration and Overheating

Becoming dehydrated is easy, especially when you are active. Dehydration can cause serious problems for older adults. Severe dehydration can cause you to be hospitalized.

During activity it's normal for your body to produce heat and for you to sweat. If you are wearing the right clothing and the temperature and humidity are not excessive, the sweat will evaporate off your skin to cool your body. If you are exercising in hot and humid conditions, you will sweat more than normal. You must replace the water that you are losing to avoid becoming dehydrated. As you get older, you will not be able to rely on feeling thirsty to remind you to drink water.

Dehydration can lead to overheating and heat stroke. Both are serious conditions. See the warning signs of overheating and heat stroke on page 78. Dehydration can also cause constipation, make kidney problems worse, and cause blood pressure to drop.

Taking diuretics ("water pills"), antihistamines, antidepression medicines, and other medicines can cause dehydration. Drinking caffeinated and alcoholic beverages can also cause you to lose fluid and need more water.

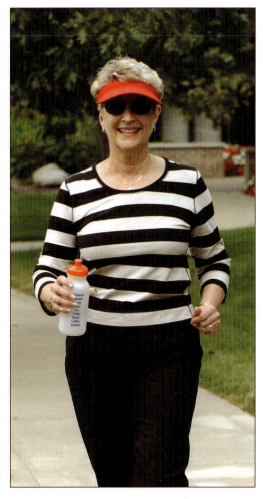

When walking outdoors in bright sunlight, don't forget your sunglasses and a sun-shielding hat that won't blow away.

Be sure to drink water throughout the day to prevent dehydration. You can tell if you are becoming dehydrated if your urine becomes dark yellow. Your goal should be to drink six to eight cups of liquids every day. Drink one cup of water before and after activity—more in hot and humid weather. If you are active for more than 30 minutes, drink another cup of water during your activity.

Plain water is the best liquid to drink. Other nonalcoholic, decaffeinated drinks, such as fruit and vegetable juices, lemonade, and low-fat or nonfat milk, count as fluids. You don't need to buy sports drinks to replace the minerals lost through sweating unless you are working hard for several hours. If you have a problem with incontinence, don't manage the problem by drinking less water. Talk to your doctor about ways to drink the water that you need and control incontinence. Give yourself time to adjust to activity in hot or humid weather or at high altitude. Also, remember to wear the right clothing for the activity that you will do.

Warning Signs of Overheating and Heat Stroke

Stop, get out of the sun, and drink water if you have any of these symptoms during activity.

- Headache
- Light-headedness or dizziness
- Confusion
- Clumsiness or stumbling
- Nausea or vomiting
- Muscle cramps
- Excess sweating or no sweating at all
- Chills

Organize Your Surroundings to Promote Activity

If you want to be active every day or nearly every day, getting organized is helpful. Action box 5.1 suggests ways in which you can arrange your surroundings to support your good intentions. You can provide yourself with visible cues or prompts that will remind you to be active at home, at work, and during leisure time. You may also need to remove some things from your surroundings that encourage you to be inactive.

Use reminders on your calendar to be active.

Action Box 5.1: Cues and Prompts for Physical Activity

Review the following suggestions about how you can remind yourself to be active. Mark the ones that might work for you. Add additional ideas that you think of in the blanks provided. Commit to trying one new cue in each area during the coming week.

At Home

____ Lay out your clothes the night before for early morning activity.

____ Keep shoes for activity in several places—the garage, the car, the van, places you visit frequently.

____ Always keep a workout bag packed and handy.

____ Wear clothes for physical activity around the house.

____ Turn off the television before or after dinner and go for a walk.

____ Don't pick up the newspaper or read the mail in the afternoon until you have gone for a walk.

____ Keep all your workout clothes in one drawer.

____ Freeze containers of water to take along on outings.

____ Post affirmations about physical activity on your bathroom mirror.

My Cues for Activity at Home

- _____

- _____

- _____

At Work

____ Schedule activity or stretch breaks during meetings at work.

____ Write on your personal calendar reminders to be active.

____ Set your watch or computer to remind you to stretch every hour.

____ Place pictures on your bulletin board of you and others engaged in physical activity.

____ Always wear comfortable shoes.

____ Keep resistance rubber bands or small dumbbells handy for a few quick repetitions.

(continued)

My Cues for Activity at Work

- ■ _____

- ■ _____

- ■ _____

During Leisure Time

____ Spend time with others who are active.

____ Always carry clothes for activity, especially shoes, in the car.

____ Request information about active vacations.

____ Make reservations at hotels that have onsite fitness facilities.

My Cues for Activity During Leisure Time

- ■ _____

- ■ _____

- ■ _____

Personal Profile

Rubin, Age 59

Rubin likes to watch television when he gets in from work. In the past when he walked in the door, his habit was to get a beer from the refrigerator, pick up the newspaper, sit in his recliner, turn on the TV with the remote control, and watch TV while his wife prepared dinner. Most nights they ate from TV trays. On some evenings Rubin didn't move from the recliner until he got up to go to bed. When he decided to try to be more active, he made a few changes in his surroundings to help support his new habit. First, he put his walking shoes in the laundry room, so that he saw them when he entered the house. He read the newspaper in the morning and then threw it away. He put a reminder on the refrigerator to walk and kept a bottle filled with cold water to take along on his walk. He filled his recliner with throw pillows so that he couldn't sit down, and he gave his wife the remote control. And they agreed to walk for 30 minutes before eating at the dining table. Rubin still enjoys watching television for a while in the evening. He is thinking about buying a stationary cycle so that he can ride while watching TV, but he's not ready to do it just yet. He wants to be sure that he can continue to walk after work before making such a big investment. He will track his thoughts and actions for a couple more months before making a decision.

Use Rewards for Reinforcement

Rewards can be helpful in achieving goals and sustaining new habits, especially when getting started. Typically, adults are uncomfortable giving themselves rewards. We use rewards effectively with children to reinforce positive behaviors, but we resist using them for ourselves.

The two major types of rewards are intangible rewards and tangible ones. Intangible rewards don't cost anything. In fact, many people say that being active (feeling and looking good) is its own reward. In many ways, tangible rewards are easier to plan for than intangible ones. Everyone likes to get a gift. You know best what is likely to mean the most to you. A reward doesn't have to cost much, but it should be special. The gift to yourself shouldn't be something that you are likely to buy regardless of your goal. If the reward is something that requires more money than you have at the time, you can earn the money for the reward. Put aside a small amount of money each day you achieve your short-term goal. Some people pay themselves for doing physical tasks that they would have to pay others to do, such as housecleaning, washing the car, painting a room, or cutting the grass.

Support from others is extremely helpful when you are trying to increase your activity. Agree to share a reward with another person who is supporting your physical activity goal. See the list of ideas for rewards involving others. Complete action box 5.2 to identify intangible and tangible rewards to reinforce your efforts to be more active. These questions may help you decide on rewards that are likely to work for you.

- What would be a nice present to receive from a friend or family member?
- If you had a small amount of extra money, how would you spend it?
- What do you like to do for fun?
- What are your hobbies or major interests?
- What makes you feel really good?
- What would you hate to lose?
- Who would be proud of you for achieving your physical activity goals?

Action Box 5.2:   Rewards—What Would Appeal to You?

Here are a few ideas for rewards that have worked well for others. Mark those that appeal to you. Add your own ideas for rewards that you would like.

(continued)

Intangible Rewards

_____ Put your daily physical activity goal on your "To do" list each day. Check off the goal when you've completed it. You'll enjoy the feelings of accomplishment. Make the reward more tangible by putting a colorful sticker on your calendar for the days that you achieve your goal.

_____ Use affirmations to give yourself a compliment for being active. You might tell yourself, "I look and feel great!" "I'm proud of myself for staying active," or "I'm having a wonderful time."

_____ Write a positive statement about your physical activity in your journal or on your personal calendar.

_____ Give yourself the gift of time. Put aside 10 minutes for each day that you accomplish your goal. At the end of the week, you'll have at least an hour that you can spend doing something just for you, such as browsing at a flea market or museum or working on a craft.

I would also like the following intangible rewards:

_____

_____

_____

Tangible Rewards

_____ Have a pedicure, manicure, massage, or facial.

_____ Choose a new perfume or cologne.

_____ Buy bubble bath and enjoy soaking in the tub.

_____ Buy something small to wear that reminds you of the goal you achieved, such as a pen, scarf, tie, belt, or bracelet.

_____ Go to a concert, play, or movie.

_____ Buy flowers or a plant for your home or office.

_____ Plant a small tree or shrub in your yard and watch it grow.

_____ If you like tools or gadgets, buy something to use in the kitchen or workshop.

_____ Hang a birdhouse or wind chimes in a spot that is visible to you.

_____ If you are raising your grandchildren, hire a babysitter for a few hours. Spend the time doing something for yourself.

_____ Get the car detailed.

I would also like the following tangible rewards:

_____

_____

_____

Rewards planned in advance work best, so fit the reward to your goal. In the beginning, you may choose to reward yourself for working toward a short-term goal rather than achieving your overall goal. In the next section, you will have an opportunity to set a short-term goal and establish a meaningful reward. Later you will use rewards as part of your long-term plan for staying active.

Ideas for Rewards Involving Others

Here are a few ideas for rewards that you can share:

- Take dancing lessons, stay overnight at a bed and breakfast, go fishing or hiking—anything that you both enjoy and that doesn't sabotage your efforts to stay healthy (such as going out for burgers and beer).
- Listen for compliments from others and acknowledge them. Say, "Thank you for noticing. I'm working hard to increase my physical activity. I'm glad it shows!"
- Make long-distance phone calls to friends or family members whom you don't speak with often.
- Volunteer your services or contribute to a charity.
- Ask someone to give you positive feedback about your activity on a regular basis.

Set a Short-Term Goal to Be More Active

Use action box 5.3 to set a goal that matches your current stage of readiness for physical activity. If you are just beginning to increase your physical activity, focus on short-term goals—things that you can accomplish in a day or two (not more than a week). Because you need to do many tasks to get organized for activity, your first goals may not involve any actual physical activity. That's fine. Working toward your goal of becoming more active is what is important at this time. Review the tasks outlined in the "Chapter Checklist" at the end of each of the first four chapters for ideas for short-term goals. Also, see "Tips for Goal Setting" on the next page.

If you are already active, your goal will probably include physical activity. But if you are interested in trying a different type of activity, you will find that you must repeat many of the tasks that you used when you were first getting started. The ability to repeat the processes, skills, and stages of change is a major advantage of this approach to staying physically active over your lifetime.

Tips for Goal Setting

- Be specific when you set your goal. For example, say, "I will walk briskly for 10 minutes without stopping on four days this week."

- Make your goal challenging, but not out of reach. Ask yourself if someone else like you could achieve the goal. If your answer is yes, your goal is probably realistic.

- Write your goal on paper. Use the personal contract in action box 5.3 or write your goal on your calendar or in your journal.

- Plan to reward yourself for working toward and achieving your goal. Make the reward something that is meaningful to you.

- Consider sharing your goal with another person. Have someone sign your personal contract as a witness. Being accountable to someone helps keep you motivated. Your friend can provide support and even share a reward with you when you are successful.

Action Box 5.3: My Personal Contract

Example: Betty (Preparation Stage)

For the week of June 13 (week 1), I, Betty, will do the following tasks to increase my physical activity.

Day	What I will do
Sunday, June 13	Read an article about walking in a fitness magazine. Take an inventory of my clothing for physical activity and organize it into one drawer. Identify any items that I need to buy.
Monday, June 14	Ask Mindy (an experienced walker) to go shopping with me for walking shoes at a sporting-goods store on Thursday. Start wearing a step counter to track my current level of physical activity.
Tuesday, June 15	Record my daily steps as measured by the step counter.
Wednesday, June 16	Record my daily steps as measured by the step counter. Review my pros and cons for becoming more active.
Thursday, June 17	Record my daily steps as measured by the step counter. Shop for walking shoes with Mindy.
Friday, June 18	Try out my new walking shoes with a 10-minute walk in my neighborhood.
Saturday, June 19	Meet Mindy at the high school track. Walk together. Get tips from her about how to get started with a regular walking program. Go for coffee with Mindy to celebrate my progress this week.

When I complete the activities listed above, I will reward myself as follows: *Mindy and I will go for coffee after our walk on Saturday.*

I will involve Mindy in my plan as follows: *She will go shopping with me for walking shoes and other clothing items.*

Signed: *Betty*   Date: *June 10*

Witness: *Mindy*   Date: *June 11*

My Personal Contract

For the week of _____, I, (your name) _____

_____, will do the following tasks to increase my physical activity.

Day	What I will do
Sunday	
Monday	
Tuesday	
Wednesday	
Thursday	
Friday	
Saturday	

When I complete the activities listed above, I will reward myself as follows:

_____

_____

_____

I will involve _____ in my plan as follows:

_____

_____

_____

Signed: _____ Date:_____

Witness: _____ Date:_____

Weigh Your Pros and Cons

In chapter 2 you learned about how the pros and cons that you see for physical activity can change as you increase your physical activity. Before proceeding to the next chapter, review your pros and cons. The appendix includes a copy of the form. Count the total number of marks in each column. Look back at your responses on pages 31 and 32 compared with your responses now. Are you seeing more advantages for physical activity? Are you finding it easier to solve problems and break down barriers that have prevented you from being active in the past?

If your score for pros outweighs your score for cons, congratulations! You are on your way to becoming and staying active. If you still seem to have many cons, go back and review some of the information in chapters 1 and 3 about the benefits of physical activity, especially as you get older. The merits of physical activity are too important to ignore.

Summary

You would probably agree that just about all of us can organize our lives to be more active. Do you have what you need to get started? Have you organized your surroundings to support your physical activity habits? If you are ready, why not use what you've learned in this chapter to set a short-term goal to start working toward more activity? In this chapter, we covered selection and fitting of shoes, choosing clothes for activity, and caring for your feet—steps that you may need to take as you begin to lead your new active lifestyle. Remember that you don't have to do structured exercise if you are not ready. If you need more time to get organized, then your short-term goals may not include physical activity. If you think that you might be ready to move toward a more formal program, the next chapter will help you lay the foundation for your fitness plan. Don't forget to reward yourself as you make progress toward your activity goals. You know that rewards work for kids. They work for adults too.

Chapter Checklist

Following are some ways in which you can apply what you have learned in this chapter to your daily life. Over the next few days and weeks try to do as many of these activities as possible.

- ❑ Obtain a comfortable, good-fitting pair of shoes and appropriate clothing for the activity that you plan to do. Check your shoes to see how they wear and whether you need shoes with special features. If your shoes are worn out, replace them.

- ❑ Consider your step counter part of your regular attire. Wear it every day to monitor your overall physical activity. Your average steps per day should increase some every week.

❑ Think of ways to give yourself cues to be active at home, at work, and during leisure time. Commit to trying one new cue in each area during the next week.

❑ Write a personal contract to achieve a short-term goal to be more active. Your contract should be for one week.

❑ Think about rewards that you will give yourself now (short term) and in the future (long term). Be sure that the rewards are meaningful to you.

❑ Continue to review your list of pros and cons for physical activity. Your list of pros should be getting longer, and your list of cons should be getting shorter.

❑ Practice affirmations to motivate yourself to be active. See page 82 for affirmations to try or write some of your own. Affirmations will increase your confidence that you can stay active for a lifetime.

Word Search

See if you can find 10 important words from this chapter in the grid that follows. Words appear forward and backward in rows, columns, and diagonals. The solution is shown on page 231.

```
U A E M Y J C I Z T P D E V V
G N I T T I F L L E W T K P V
U E O T P D I E V X X G O Q S
W Z H I B M Z W B U D J R B H
J X Z A T I S L A O G L T H O
C S G E N A T H M D J G S E E
N D J A L A R U E F Z S T G S
L W G O I U N D L R T B A A F
J R O S A E B K Y A M G E U K
O S B D E M N E L H Y U H E U
E D K N M U F W J V E E V I J
Y L Y J I J C I C W P D R A A
J T T K X L R E W A R D S S J
W R P M Y I K D X X I Q B U E
Y X G W X B R A F X C D Z R N
```

Cues	Layers	Rewards
Dehydration	Loose	Shoes
Goals	Organize	Well-fitting
Heat stroke		

Explore Aerobic Fitness

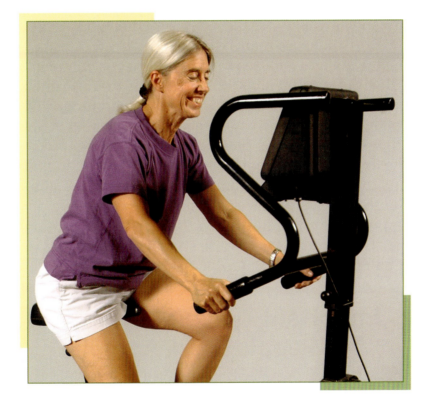

In This Chapter

❑ Recall the difference between lifestyle physical activity and structured exercise.

❑ Know the types of fitness that are most important for people after age 50.

❑ Explore walking, swimming, water activities, or stationary cycling.

❑ Repeat the Readiness to Change Questionnaire.

Most of what we have presented in this book to this point is about lifestyle physical activity. Lifestyle activity includes taking the stairs, walking to do errands, and working in your yard—all the ways in which you are active in your everyday life. Although you do most of these activities at low to moderate levels (you don't get out of breath and sweaty), they can help you maintain a good level of overall health and fitness. If you choose, you can do enough of this type of physical activity to benefit your health. Your goal should be to be active through lifestyle pursuits at least 30 minutes every day or nearly every day. You don't have to do all the activity at one time. For example, doing 10 minutes of activity three times over the course of a day would meet this goal. A major advantage of lifestyle physical activity is that you can do it almost any place and any time. You can work it in throughout the day. You don't have to change clothes, go to a special place, or take a shower when you are done. Lifestyle physical activity involves no real costs.

Remember that a slight difference exists between *physical activity* and *exercise*. Physical activity includes all movements that use energy—grooming, housekeeping chores, dancing, gardening, swimming, climbing stairs, cycling, and taking the dog for a walk. Because movement is involved, even standing (rather than sitting) is physical activity.

Structured exercise is a type of physical activity that includes walking, jogging, group fitness classes, swimming, cycling, lifting weights, stretching, yoga, and all active sports. Structured exercise is repetitive physical activity done to improve physical fitness. In this chapter, we'll start to look at some forms of structured exercise and, specifically, at types of structured exercise that can improve your aerobic fitness.

Important Types of Fitness for People After Age 50

Physical fitness is the overall ability of the body to perform physical work. Physical fitness is what happens in your body because of physical activity or exercise. You must be physically active (the action) to achieve a good level of physical fitness (the goal).

There are several types of physical fitness. This book focuses on the types of fitness that are important for your health and function as you get older. These include aerobic fitness, muscle fitness, joint flexibility, balance, and body composition. Even if you're not quite ready to tackle all these types of fitness, stay with us! The activities in this chapter will help you decide which types of fitness you'll want to work toward.

- **Aerobic fitness.** The word *aerobic* means "with oxygen." Your muscles (including your heart muscle) need oxygen to work. When you are aerobically fit, your heart, lungs, and blood vessels are in shape and can deliver oxygen to your muscles quickly and effectively. Fit people are less likely to become tired from everyday activities. They also have lower rates of heart disease, high blood pressure, stroke, obesity, type 2 diabetes, and some cancers. And they are more likely to remain independent into old age.

- **Muscle fitness.** *Muscle fitness* includes muscle strength and muscle endurance. As you grow older, muscle fitness is as important as aerobic fitness to the quality of your life and your health. *Muscle strength* is the amount of effort your muscles can exert at one time. Strength is required for movements as simple as raising your arm to dry or comb your hair or lifting your fork to put food in your mouth. Muscle strength can become a problem during the later years if decades of inactivity have caused you to lose muscle.

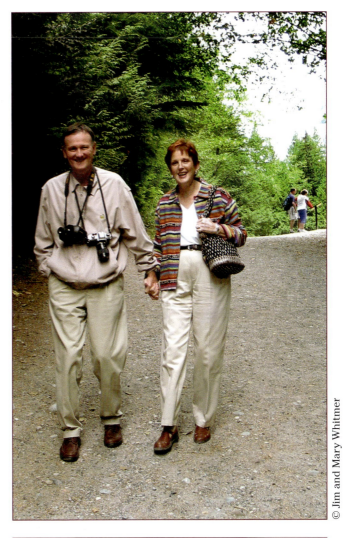

A high level of aerobic fitness makes it easier to perform routine tasks, such as walking, shopping, or sightseeing while on vacation.

Complete action box 6.1 to see whether you have already lost some muscle strength. Sophisticated, modern screening tests such CAT scans or MRIs show that many inactive older adults have little muscle left in their arms and legs. Fortunately, physical activity can help you regain muscle strength, no matter how old you are. Studies have shown that even at ages beyond 90 years people can build muscle tissue, increase strength, and become stronger.

Muscle endurance, the ability to continue to perform a task repeatedly, is related to muscle strength. If you are doing a task that requires a high percentage of your muscle strength, you will not be able to do the task for long. For example, if you are fit enough to climb three flights of stairs without pausing, climbing one flight would be easy. If you lost most of the muscle strength in your legs, however, you would have to stop and rest after every step or two.

Action Box 6.1:   Have You Lost Muscle Strength?

Mark any of the following tasks that are difficult for you to do one time.

_____ Pick up a small child

_____ Carry two bags of groceries from your car to the kitchen

_____ Climb a flight of stairs

_____ Move a piece of heavy furniture

_____ Get up from a low chair or sofa without using your arms

List other difficult tasks here:

_____

_____

If any of these tasks are difficult for you, you may have lost a lot of muscle strength. Unless you do something to reverse it, the decline in your strength will continue. You could lose more than strength. You could lose your independence! But this doesn't have to happen to you. In chapter 10 we'll show you some ways to regain your strength.

■ **Joint flexibility.** _Flexibility_ is the ability to move muscles and joints through their full range of motion. If you routinely perform stretches, you are probably still pretty flexible. Although normally not a problem for most young people, lack of joint flexibility can become limiting after decades of inactivity. Lack of flexibility in the arms and shoulders is especially common in older adults. Inflexibility can become severe enough that you find it hard to turn your head and look behind you. This problem is unimportant while you are sitting in a recliner and watching television, but it may be critical when you try to back your car out of a parking place in a crowded parking lot. As another example, loss of flexibility may make it difficult for you to tie your shoes. Many routine tasks you used to do with ease may now be difficult or impossible with declining flexibility.

Complete action box 6.2 to check your flexibility. Exercises to improve muscle strength, muscle endurance, and joint flexibility are provided in chapter 10.

Action Box 6.2:   How Flexible Are You?

Mark any of the tasks that are difficult for you to do.

_____ Bending over to tie your shoes

_____ Touching your toes

_____ Turning your head to look behind you

_____ Buttoning a blouse in the back or fastening a bra

_____ Raising your arms to dry or comb your hair

_____ Scratching your back

_____ Lying on your stomach with your head turned to one side

_____ Putting on a snug-fitting jacket

List other difficult tasks here:

_____

_____

■ **Balance.** _Balance_ is your ability to maintain your body in its upright posture while moving. Having good balance is important for many common movements, such as getting on and off the bus. You need good balance to be able to avoid falling if you trip over an object or try to grasp something that is just out of reach. Falling is the leading cause of accidental injury and death in people over age 65. Even among people in their 50s, falling causes fractures, especially in women whose bones become thinner after menopause.

Do the tests for balance described in action box 6.3. You can do specific exercises to improve balance. In general, you should do exercises to develop strong muscles in your trunk region (back and stomach), in your hips and legs, and around your ankles.

Action Box 6.3: Test Your Balance

Balance on One Foot

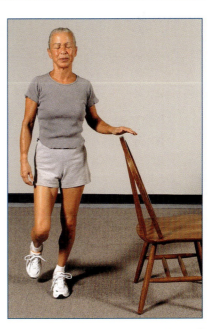

1. Stand next to a chair while performing this test or have someone assist you.

2. Stand on your right foot without holding the chair. Count to 10.

3. If you are able to keep your balance, try standing on the same foot with your eyes closed.

4. Now change to your left foot and see whether you can stand for a count of 10 with your eyes closed.

(continued)

Fill in your results:

> I was able to count to _____ while standing on my right foot.

> I was able to count to _____ while standing on my left foot.

> I was able to count to _____ while standing on my right foot with my eyes closed.

> I was able to count to _____ while standing on my left foot with my eyes closed.

> People with good balance can stand for 10 seconds on one foot without holding the chair and with their eyes closed. If you can't, you could benefit from exercises to improve your balance. See chapter 10 for balance exercises.

Forward Reach

1. Stand with your feet shoulder-width apart and your right shoulder against a wall.

2. Raise your right arm level with your shoulder and mark the spot where your fingertips touch the wall.

3. Keeping your back straight, reach forward with your right arm outstretched.

4. Measure the number of inches or centimeters that your fingertips can reach forward before you must take a step to prevent yourself from tumbling forward.

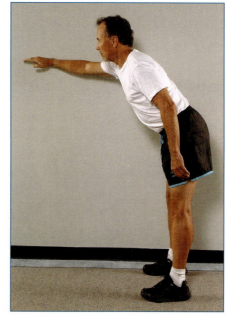

Fill in your results:

> I was able to reach forward _____ inches (centimeters) before losing my balance.

> People with good balance can reach forward at least 12 to 15 inches (30 to 38 centimeters) before they must catch themselves. If you can't, you are at increased risk of injuries from falls. See chapter 10 for exercises to improve balance and prevent falls.

■ **Body composition.** Your body composition—the ratio of fat to lean tissue—plays an important role in your health and function. Body composition is an important part of fitness for older adults. Beginning around age 30, people typically begin gaining weight at the average rate of 1 pound (0.45 kilograms) per year until about age 50 (for men) or 60 (for women). After these ages, weight usually becomes stable for a few years before beginning a gradual decline. For most people, the decline in weight in later years is caused not by loss of fat but by loss of muscle and bone. People who are overweight or underweight have more health problems than do those who maintain a normal weight.

Remember Your Youth

Your thoughts and actions related to physical activity have likely changed over time. Those of us who grew up in the 1930s to the 1950s were probably very active as children. Active play was the vocation of childhood. Unlike kids today, who watch a lot of television or spend hours at a time in front of a computer, we spent much of our out-of-school time playing outdoors. Many of our games, such as red rover and hide-and-seek, involved running. Play didn't require equipment, coaches, or referees. We created games to fit our surroundings and meet our needs at the time. Kids didn't have to be athletes to play and be active.

Think back over the decades about the types of activity that you have enjoyed. Don't limit your thoughts to what is considered traditional exercise today. Make notes about your physical activities at various ages in action box 6.4. Involve all your senses in your memories. See yourself in your mind's eye. Remember the sounds around you. How did you feel about yourself? If possible, collect old pictures of yourself engaged in physical activity and put them in places where you can see them every day.

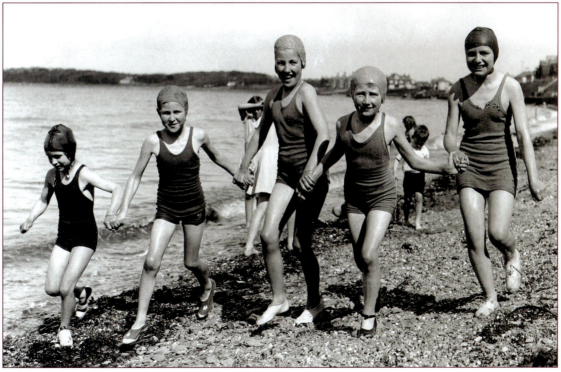

© Getty Images

Do you remember when you didn't have to be an athlete to play and be active?

Action Box 6.4: Ways in Which You Were Active in the Past

Age	Write in this space about physical activities that you enjoyed when you were younger. Tell about what the activity was, where it occurred, and who was involved.	Activities that you may have enjoyed
Before age 6		Riding a tricycle Kick ball Swinging and sliding Climbing Hide-and-seek Other games involving running Throwing and catching a ball
Ages 6 to 12		Hopscotch Jumping rope Softball Dancing lessons (tap, ballet) Gymnastics Riding a bicycle Roller skating or ice skating Horseback riding
Ages 13 to 18		Team sports, such as softball, basketball, football, or soccer Individual sports, such as tennis, golf, or wrestling Track or cross-country Hiking Fishing Social dancing Roller or ice skating Marching in the band, drill team, or pep squad Gymnastics
Ages 19 to 29		Team sports, such as softball, basketball, football, or soccer Individual sports, such as tennis, golf, or wrestling Hiking Fishing Social dancing Roller skating or ice skating Playing with young children Snow skiing or water skiing

Personal Profiles

Jack, Age 70

Jack was an outstanding athlete in high school. He lettered in several sports and earned a track scholarship for college. Although he can't run or jog because of an old knee injury, he still thinks of himself as an athlete. He enjoys an active retirement—playing golf, fishing, playing with his grandchildren, and traveling with his wife. Jack was one of the best dancers in his high school class, and he met his wife at a dance. They go out dancing frequently and are usually the best dancers on the floor.

Sara, Age 64

Sara was an active teenager. She didn't play any sports, but she was a majorette with the marching band. Marching up and down the football field for several hours each week was a common activity for about six months of the year during her high school days. When the band was not marching, Sara stayed active by practicing baton-twirling routines almost every day. Recently, Sara enrolled in a group fitness class. She found the steps and movements similar to the routines that she performed as a teenager. Now, she also enjoys walking on the track at a local high school. Sometimes the band is practicing while she is walking. Seeing the band and hearing the music bring back memories of her teenage years and keep her motivated.

Aerobic Physical Activities

All types of fitness are important. We will discuss physical activities to improve aerobic fitness first.

Many people ask, "What type of aerobic activity is best? What type should I do?" No one type of aerobic activity is best. As you can see in the following list of popular aerobic activities, numerous types of aerobic activities are available for you to choose from. Choose one that you think you will enjoy and try it.

- Brisk walking
- Bench stepping or stair climbing
- Hiking
- Jogging
- Swimming
- Water aerobics
- Rowing
- Group fitness classes
- Cycling

In this chapter we are going to focus on three aerobic activities that are popular with people over age 50—walking, swimming or water aerobics, and stationary cycling. We will discuss sports and recreational activities in chapter 10.

Walking for Exercise

Walking is the most popular aerobic activity with people of all ages, not just those over age 50. If you haven't been active in the past, walking is an excellent way to get started with exercise. If you have been active in the past, perhaps as a jogger or runner, walking may be your exercise of choice as you get older. Walking for exercise and sport has much to recommend it. Some of the best reasons to walk and various types of walking are described next. The types of walking differ depending on your purpose, pace, and posture (the length of your stride and how you hold your arms).

Reasons to Walk

- Walking is easy to do. No special skills are required to get started.

- You don't need any special equipment, except a comfortable, good-fitting pair of shoes.

- You can do it almost anytime and anywhere—outdoors or indoors at a mall, gymnasium, or airport.

- Because walking is convenient and easy to do, you are more likely to stay with it. The dropout rate for walking is lower than it is for any other type of exercise.

- Walking is a safe, low-impact activity. The impact of walking is one-fifth that of jogging. You're not likely to be injured.

- You can increase your intensity as you improve your fitness level.

- Walking is a weight-bearing activity that can help build strong leg muscles and bones.

- You can burn more energy by walking faster or longer.

- You can walk alone or with a partner or group.

- You can participate in special walking events and competitions.

- Walking can help reduce stress.

Types of Walking

Believe it or not, there are many different types of walking to choose from. See which one appeals to you.

Standing and intermittent walking—Cooking, office work, and grooming tasks are activities that involve mostly standing around and a little walking. Besides walking for physical activity, try to be on your feet for at least an hour a day.

Strolling or casual walking (30 minutes per mile or 19 minutes per kilometer)—Activities such as shopping or walking with small children are considered low intensity, but they burn more energy (calories or kilojoules) than sitting or standing does.

Functional walking (20 to 30 minutes per mile or about 13 to 19 minutes per kilometer)—This type of walking gets you where you're going or allows you to perform a task. Functional walking burns some energy and may provide the break that you need in a stressful situation.

Brisk walking (15 to 20 minutes per mile or 9 to 13 minutes per kilometer)—You'll get significant health benefits from this type of walking, especially if you do it for a minimum of 30 minutes a day.

Striding or power walking (12 to 15 minutes per mile or about 7 to 9 minutes per kilometer)—With this form of walking, you increase the length of your stride and usually pump your arms.

Techniques and Tips for Walking

Offering pointers on walking may seem odd because walking is something that you already know how to do and

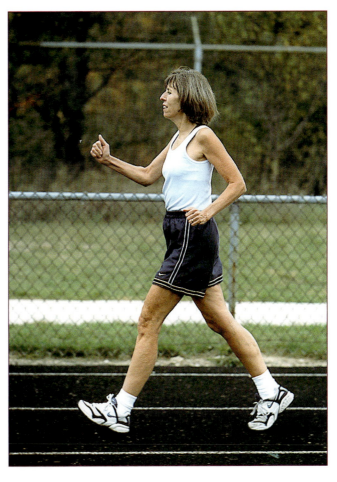

With power walking, the extra effort of the arms and legs increases the intensity and burns more energy.

do regularly. But when you are walking for your health and fitness, a few reminders may be helpful:

- Stand upright with your head level and shoulders relaxed. Think tall.

- Reach out your leg with your knee, heel, and toe pointed forward. Use smooth movements, rolling from heel to toe.

- Try to walk without carrying anything in your hands so that your arms can swing naturally at your sides in opposition to your legs. Carry your keys, identification, a small amount of money, and other necessary items in a small pack that you can strap around your waist.

- Start slowly and then pick up your pace by taking quicker and longer steps. Be careful not to compromise your upright posture or smooth, easy movements.

- For a pace up to 4 miles per hour, or 15 minutes per mile (6.4 kilometers per hour, or about 9 minutes per kilometer), walk with your body erect and arms fully extended in an easy swing. As you increase your pace, change to a bent-arm swing with your arms at a 90-degree angle. Make a loose fist with your hands. Keep your elbows close to your body.

- Breathe in and out naturally, rhythmically, and deeply.

Variations of Walking

You can add variety to a walking program in many ways. One way is to change your pace or intensity. For example, do a few minutes of power walking and then do a few minutes of regular brisk walking. Walking in a swimming pool is another way to stimulate your walking program. The water adds resistance to increase the intensity of the exercise. Walking uphill is one of the most natural ways to increase the intensity of walking without increasing the pace. If hilly terrain is not available, you can use

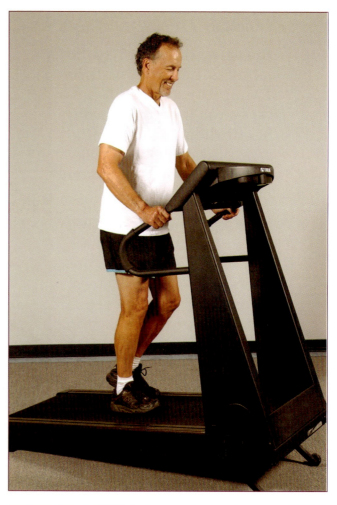

Hold the handles only as long as needed to gain your balance.

a treadmill or stair-climbing machine to get a similar result. See safety tips for walking outdoors next.

Treadmills, stair-climbers, and other cardiovascular machines are commonly available in health clubs and fitness centers. An advantage of these machines is that you can perform your exercise at an exact level of intensity for a specified period. Because you are indoors, you don't have to be concerned about weather or other environmental conditions. Some machines allow you to monitor your heart rate and calculate the number of calories or kilojoules burned during your exercise session.

When walking on a motorized treadmill or stair-climbing machine, concentrate on maintaining good balance and rhythm. Hold the bar or handle only as long as necessary to gain your balance. Then let go of the bar and walk or step without holding on. Look straight ahead and increase or decrease the speed as needed. If you must hold the bar, you should realize that your arms are not doing any work. You are working at a lower intensity than you would be if you didn't hold on.

Safety Tips for Outdoor Activity

Walking is one of the safest exercises you can do. If you are walking outdoors, however, taking precautions is wise. These precautions are appropriate for any outdoor activity that you may do:

- Carry identification or write your name and phone number on the inside of your shoe. Carry medical information if necessary.

- Do not wear expensive jewelry or carry valuables.

- Carry water with you or plan a water stop if you are going to be out for an extended period. See the information about dehydration in chapter 5.

- If you want to wear headphones, use the type that doesn't block noise. You need to be able to hear cars and other potential dangers.

- Dress appropriately for the weather. Check the forecast if you're planning to be outdoors for an extended time.

- Use extra caution if you are outdoors in very cold (below freezing) and windy or very hot (above 90 degrees Fahrenheit, or 32 degrees Celsius) and humid weather.

- Avoid areas where snow, ice, or wet leaves may accumulate.

- Avoid midday heat, use sunscreen, and wear a hat.

(continued)

Safety Tips for Outdoor Activity *(continued)*

- Consider air quality—pollution from cars, pollen (if you have allergies), and ozone warnings. Early morning is often the best time of day for outdoor activities.

- Walk in a familiar area and plan your routes. Choose routes that include the fewest number of crossings.

- Be careful when crossing at traffic lights where right turns against red lights are permitted. Use crosswalks as much as possible.

- Stay alert to dangerous situations. Avoid unpopulated areas, deserted streets, and overgrown trails. Also, avoid poorly lighted areas, parked cars, and unleashed dogs.

- Walk against traffic so that you see oncoming vehicles. Be alert at intersections for changing lights and curbs. Wear reflective material if you are out before dawn or after dark.

- Ignore verbal harassment. Look directly at strangers but keep your distance and keep moving.

- Respect your intuition. If you feel unsafe, honor that feeling and get away from trouble.

- Don't walk, jog, or cycle outdoors after dark, unless you are in an off-road, well-lighted area. Even if you wear reflective clothing and equipment, being out on the road when it is dark is dangerous. Also, if your night vision is poor, you may be less able to see cracks and potholes in the road surface or other obstacles on the pathway.

- Walk with a partner. If walking alone, tell someone your route and expected time of return.

Water Activities

Water activities are popular with people over age 50. Moving in water is easier than moving on land. People with arthritis feel less pain in their joints when exercising in water. Exercising in warm water may be even more comfortable.

Swimming

Swimming is an excellent exercise for overall fitness. Besides strengthening your heart and lungs, swimming keeps other muscles (shoulders, back, arms, legs) strong. As a survival skill, swimming gives you confidence to do many other recreational activities such as sailing, canoeing or kayaking, and snorkeling.

The amount of calories or kilojoules that you burn while swimming depends on the stroke you use, how fast you swim, your swimming skills, and your body composition (body fatness). A poor swimmer is less efficient and burns more energy than a skilled swimmer does.

If you didn't learn to swim as a child, it's not too late to learn. Many people over age 50 take swimming lessons for the first time in their lives. The principal disadvantage of swimming is that you need a pool, or possibly a natural body of water, that is convenient to use. If you're interested in swimming laps, you'll probably need to find a standard 25-yard (or 25-meter) pool.

Many schools, universities, hotels, community recreation centers, and health or fitness clubs have swimming facilities. In parts of some countries where the summers are hot, many homes have backyard swimming pools. Although home pools may not be suited for swimming laps, you can still use them for water activities. Many residential communities have neighborhood pools.

Reasons to Swim

Swimming offers numerous advantages:

- Swimming uses most major muscle groups—shoulders, back, arms, legs.

- Swimming provides more upper-body exercise than walking, jogging, or cycling does.

- Swimming is a nonimpact and non-weight-bearing exercise. It's easy on the joints, which is especially important if you have problems because of injuries, arthritis, or osteoporosis.

- Despite its gentle cushioning, water provides 12 times more resistance than air does, so you can burn a large amount of energy, even with slow swimming.

- The risk of stress fracture is nil.

- You can participate at various levels of skill.

- If an indoor or heated pool is available, you can swim year round.

- Many hotels have pools, which makes exercising easy when you travel.

- Good swimmers can enjoy other water activities, such as sailing, canoeing, and snorkeling.

Besides a swimsuit, you might consider these pieces of swimming equipment:

Swim cap—to keep your hair relatively dry and out of your face

Goggles—to protect your eyes from chlorine in the pool water and from debris in open water, and to allow you to open your eyes to see underwater

Waterproof watch—to time your exercise session

Kickboard—to support your upper body while kicking

Hand paddles—to increase arm and shoulder strength

Swim fins—to increase ankle and leg strength

Pull buoy—to support your feet while using only your arms to swim

Water toys (beach balls, volleyballs)—to add variety and fun

Water Aerobics

You can do other aerobic exercises in water besides swimming. These exercises provide a good transition for you while you are learning your strokes. You can also alternate some of these activities with swimming laps. Try these exercises in water that is waist to chest deep.

- Walk through the water moving your arms in a swim stroke motion.

- Walk or skip across the pool (forward and backward). Use the wall, a kickboard, or a rope for balance, if needed.

- Jog in place, either bringing the knees as high as possible or kicking the feet toward the buttocks. Travel forward, backward, or from side to side. Make a one-quarter turn every eight counts. Add hand weights (holding them underwater) to any of these moves.

- Kick to the front or sides, swinging the legs (straight legs).

- Kick to the front or sides, bringing the knee up (like kick boxing) and kicking forward.

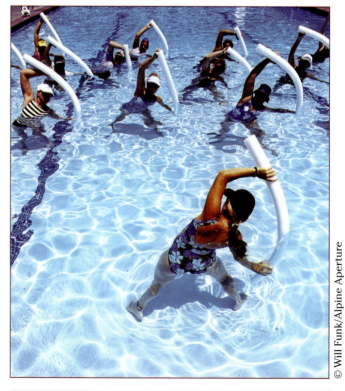

© Will Funk/Alpine Aperture

Water aerobics can help you maintain aerobic fitness.

- Kick to the sides, bringing the knee up and then kicking out ("cowboy kicks").

- Kick flutter style, hanging on the pool wall (face any direction) or while holding hand weights underwater.

- Kick traveling forward or backyard (like kickball kicks).

- Throw balls or play games while in the water.

Techniques and Tips for Water Activities

Feeling anxious or afraid of the water is the greatest problem that most people must overcome. You must learn to relax in the water, immersing yourself in it and moving through it. Trying to stay on top of the water tires you and makes you feel tense.

If you don't know how to swim, take lessons to learn to swim correctly. Group and private lessons are available in most communities. Knowing a variety of swimming skills will make you more confident and comfortable in the water. There are at least five basic strokes to choose from: elementary backstroke, front crawl, back crawl, breaststroke, and sidestroke. Learn the stroke or strokes that are most enjoyable for you.

Always follow these safety tips while swimming or doing any type of water activity:

- Swim in a pool that has a comfortable water temperature (83 to 88 degrees Fahrenheit, or 28 to 31 degrees Celsius). Cool water can contribute to stiffness, especially if you have arthritis. Get wet gradually so that your body can adjust to the cooler water temperature.

- Learn to float face down and practice floating on your back so that you know you can rest any time you need to.

- Learn to feel comfortable with your face in the water. Submerge with your eyes open. Wear goggles if the chlorine bothers your eyes.

- Practice bobbing to learn to control your breathing.

- Take time to do a few easy stretches before and after your swim. Flexibility is necessary for making full strokes.

- Learn to use the ratings of perceived exertion (RPE), discussed in chapter 9, to monitor how hard you are working while swimming. Taking your pulse in water is more difficult than taking it on land, so your pulse rate estimate is likely to be inaccurate.

- Be courteous to other swimmers if you are sharing lanes in a lap pool.

- If you have an allergy to chlorine in pool water or if you develop one, use goggles, a nose clip, or a mask to protect your eyes and nose.

- Be aware of the depth of the water and any potential hazards before going in. Know where the pool ladder or steps are. Swimming in open water has its own set of risks, including rocks, pollution, currents, and sudden changes in water temperature.

■ Never swim alone, regardless of your skill level.

■ Vary your strokes to avoid pain from overusing joints in the foot, knee, or shoulders.

■ Shower with soap and water immediately after swimming and apply a moisturizing lotion to your skin to prevent excessive dryness caused by pool chemicals.

■ Use an over-the-counter drug containing acetic acid if you get excess water in your ear canal (called swimmer's ear). If pain persists, see your doctor.

■ Drink water frequently, as you would with other types of exercise. Although you are surrounded by water, you still need to replace lost fluids. Because the water is washing away your perspiration and cooling your skin, you likely aren't aware of being dehydrated. Take your water bottle to the pool if a water fountain is not close by.

■ Wear water shoes or sandals around the pool and in other wet areas of a fitness center. Be especially careful to avoid slipping on wet surfaces.

Stationary Cycling

You probably enjoyed riding a bicycle when you were a child, although you didn't think of it as exercise. More likely, cycling was a major mode of transportation for you and your friends, even into your teenage years.

For adults, especially those over age 50, cycling is an excellent aerobic exercise. It requires only a minimum fitness and skill level. Because some barriers are associated with outdoor cycling (the expense of the bicycle, the dangers of the road and traffic, and the skills required to handle the bicycle and use the gears efficiently), we are going to focus on stationary cycling first. Additional reasons to use a stationary cycle are listed on the next page.

Obviously, cycling is more efficient than walking. To burn the same amount of energy (that is, calories or kilojoules), you must pedal a greater distance than you would have to walk. In general, you have to cycle about three to four times as far to burn the same amount of energy as you would by walking.

If you choose to cycle outdoors, go to parks or neighborhoods with bike paths. Go with the flow of the traffic and obey all signs. Wear a helmet that fits properly. Have your bike fitted with a water bottle holder and stop often to drink if you are riding for more than 30 minutes.

Types of Stationary Cycles

Stationary cycles are common pieces of cardiovascular equipment in health clubs and fitness centers. You can buy a stationary cycle to use at home, but we don't advise buying one until you are sure that you will enjoy this type of exercise and will stay with it. Too many pieces of home exercise equipment become expensive clothes racks. We'll discuss buying home exercise equipment later in the book. For now, if you are interested in trying stationary cycling, find a fitness center that has equipment that you can use on a trial basis.

There are several types of stationary cycles for individual use and for spinning classes. Some are similar to the bicycles designed for use on paved surfaces. These cycles are popular with those who also enjoy outdoor cycling at a fast pace. Many stationary cycles now have wide seats.

Another type of stationary cycle, called a dual-action cycle, has handlebars that move, allowing you to pump the arms as well as pedal with the legs. Dual-action cycles may use a fan that cools you while you exercise. Compared with standard bicycles, dual-action cycles use more muscle groups and provide better overall fitness.

A third type, called a recumbent cycle, has a chairlike seat that can be more comfortable than the seat on a conventional cycle, especially if you have back problems. Recumbent cycles work the hamstring muscles more than upright or dual-action cycles do. Recumbent cycles are now outselling other types of stationary cycles.

An exercise machine similar to a recumbent cycle is the Nu-Step recumbent stepper. The recumbent stepper works the front and back of the thighs and the calf muscles with a stepping rather than revolving motion.

To gauge the proper fit when you're sitting in the saddle of a cycle or recumbent stepper, adjust the seat so that your knee has only a slight bend when your foot is at the bottom of the pedal arc or step motion. Most bikes let you vary the pedaling resistance to regulate the intensity of your workout by twisting a knob or selecting a prescribed program. Monitors record your speed, distance, time, and sometimes heart rate and calories or kilojoules burned.

Reasons to Use a Stationary Cycle or Recumbent Stepper

You get an excellent aerobic workout.

You can exercise indoors at times that are convenient for you.

You don't have to worry about traffic, pollution, safety, or weather.

You can read, watch TV, or listen to music while you exercise.

Both offer non-weight-bearing exercise, so they may be easier on your joints than walking or other weight-bearing exercise.

Techniques and Tips for Cycling

Follow these tips when cycling for a safe and enjoyable ride:

- Warm up by pedaling easily for three to five minutes with low resistance. Cool down the same way.

- Pedal with a circular, spinning motion. If you use toe clips, you can pull up on one pedal as you push down on the other. Most people apply too much force on the downstroke and ease up on the upstroke. Focus less on the push-pull motion and concentrate on the roundness of your pedaling until it becomes second nature.

- Keep your feet soft on the pedals. Let your muscles do the work. Don't put all the pressure on your feet.

- Don't pedal too slowly. Your legs will quickly feel heavy. If you pedal too fast, you will expend most of your energy just fanning the pedals.

- Choose the right resistance to keep your cadence smooth and steady. At first, you'll probably find that a cadence of 60 to 70 revolutions per minute (rpm) is as fast as you can go. With practice, you should be able to spin comfortably at a brisk cadence of about 90 rpm. Larger people may opt for slightly slower cadences (80 to 85 rpm), and smaller people may find that spinning at 95 to 100 rpm is comfortable. To determine your pedaling rate, count the number of pedal revolutions you turn in 15 seconds and multiply by four.

Do You Know?

When exercising indoors on a treadmill, stationary cycle, or recumbent stepper, your body temperature will rise at a more rapid rate than it will when exercising outdoors (even at the same temperature). Outside, air moving across your body provides a cooling effect. You should expect to perspire more when exercising on machines indoors, so you may want to place a fan nearby. Also, remember to drink plenty of water if you perspire heavily.

Choose One Type of Aerobic Activity

Now that you have had a chance to explore some of the more popular aerobic exercises, choose one that you'd like to try. Answering the questions in action box 6.5 will help you decide which is best for you. All are excellent activities. Over time, you can try them all, but for now settle on one.

Action Box 6.5: Which Aerobic Activity Will You Choose?

Consider these aerobic activities: walking, walking on a treadmill, hiking, group fitness class, swimming, water aerobics, stationary cycling, and recumbent stepping.

Answer the following questions for the various types of aerobic activity. The more yes answers you give, the better that activity is likely to be for you at this time.

- Do you have a convenient place to do this type of exercise?
- If you need special equipment, is it available to you?
- If there is a cost, can you afford it?
- If you need special skills to be able to do the exercise, can you learn them?
- Can you do the exercise with a partner or group (if that is important to you)?
- Do you think that you would enjoy the exercise?

Which type of aerobic activity will you try? _____

Why? _____

_____

_____

_____

Repeat the Readiness to Change Questionnaire

We introduced the Readiness to Change Questionnaire at the beginning of this book (see pages 2-3) so that you could mark your starting point on your way to regular physical activity. How far have you come? Has what you learned so far caused you to think seriously about your physical activity level? Have you taken steps to prepare for physical activity? Have you started to do some physical activity, even if you aren't active on most days? Have you progressed to the point that you are regularly active?

Take a few minutes to complete the Readiness to Change Questionnaire again. Remember that there are no right or wrong answers. Your responses will suggest that you are in one of the five stages of readiness for changing your physical activity habits. Knowing your stage of readiness will help you focus on the skills and strategies that will keep you moving forward.

Have you progressed at least one stage since you started reading this book? If you started in precontemplation, contemplation, or preparation and have progressed at least one stage in less than 30 days, you have an excellent chance of being successful with your physical activity program. If you are now in the action or maintenance stage, congratulations!

If you are having difficulty making progress, go back and review some of the key concepts and skills from earlier chapters. Table 6.1 will help you

Table 6.1   Quick Reference Guide

Topic	Location
THINKING AND FEELING SKILLS	
Becoming more knowledgeable:	
• Health benefits of regular physical activity	Table 1.3, page 7
• Questions for your doctor about physical activity	Action box 1.4, pages 17-18
• How physical activity affects weight control	Page 11
• Being active with special conditions	Table 3.1, pages 45-48
Building confidence:	
• Analyze past successes to change	Action box 2.1, pages 23-24
• Weigh your pros and cons	Action box 2.6, pages 31-32
• Affirmations to try	Action box 3.3, page 49
Thinking differently:	
• Evaluating positive and negative forces	Action box 1.5, page 19
• Substituting rational for irrational thoughts	Action box 2.4, page 28
• Identifying the excuse	Action box 2.5, pages 29-30
Recognizing cues:	
• Keep track of your thoughts and actions	Action box 3.4. pages 50-51
• Cues and prompts for physical activity	Action box 5.1, pages 79-80
Setting goals:	
• Tips for goal setting	Page 84
• My personal contract	Action box 5.3, pages 84-85
DOING AND ACTING SKILLS	
Monitoring progress:	
• Readiness to change questionnaire	Action box 1.1, pages 2-3
• How many steps do you take each day?	Action box 4.1, page 56
• Weigh your pros and cons	Action box 2.6, pages 31-32
Managing time:	
• Personal time study	Action box 4.2, pages 57-58
• Consider your commitments	Action box 4.3, pages 60-61
• What I will do to achieve balance in my life	Action box 4.4, pages 62-63
• My ways to fit in fitness	Action box 4.5, page 66
Rewarding myself:	
• Rewards—What would appeal to you?	Action box 5.2, pages 81-83
• Ideas for rewards involving others	Page 83

find the information you need quickly. Skills are organized into two groups: thinking and feeling skills, and doing and acting skills. Both types of skills are important.

Stay positive and you will continue to progress. Remember that becoming active takes skill power as well as willpower.

Summary

In this chapter, we have discussed the types of fitness that are most important for people over age 50. We also suggested three types of activities for improving your aerobic fitness—walking, water activities, and stationary cycling. Walking is an ideal type of exercise. If you are already walking, try swimming, water aerobics, or stationary cycling. Each of these activities has much to recommend it. Thousands of older adults enjoy these activities every day. In a later chapter, you will learn how to develop an aerobic fitness program of your own. We will provide a model program for you to follow to get started with aerobic exercise or to modify a program that you are already doing. But before you start to develop an aerobic fitness program, you should think about where you will do your activity. As you will see in the next chapter, you have many possibilities to explore.

Chapter Checklist

Following are some ways in which you can apply what you have learned in this chapter to your daily life. Over the next few days and weeks try to do as many of these activities as possible.

❏ Do the self-assessments to determine your strength, flexibility, and balance. If you need to improve in any of these areas, this book will help.

❏ Think about the types of aerobic activity you would like to do. We suggest walking, treadmill walking, swimming, water aerobics, stationary cycling, or recumbent stepping. Decide on one type to try first.

❏ Continue to wear your step counter to monitor the physical activity that you get through your daily routine. Is your number of average steps per day increasing?

❏ Repeat the Readiness to Change Questionnaire. If you are having difficulty becoming more active, review the concepts and skills in earlier chapters. Keep thinking about physical activity and about yourself as an active person.

❏ Remember to say affirmations to yourself.

Word Search

See if you can find 10 important words from this chapter in the grid that follows. Words appear forward and backward in rows, columns, and diagonals. The solution is shown on page 231.

```
Y P P N V Y X A Q Y R Y V O J
L T N F L H W O K S E W A Y M
G N I L C Y C U Z B T I U I D
Z O K L H V F A Y M A E O B Q
E P S W I M M I N G W C Z B M
C A S E O B I Q H U W N B M M
V U E D L S I T Q A Y A A X V
H C L R Q C G X L B R R L I C
M I Z Y O N S K E Y G U A N K
F K J I E B I U N L L D N N H
S E R R C N I S M E F N C C T
D S T A G I L C Y H F E E Z B
B S S L G Z S Q K K T L H F K
X Y G N W H V G M C T Z I Z Z
L L C O O A H O V U O L P G R
```

Aerobic Flexibility Swimming
Balance Muscle Walking
Cycling Strength Water
Endurance

Find Places to Be Active

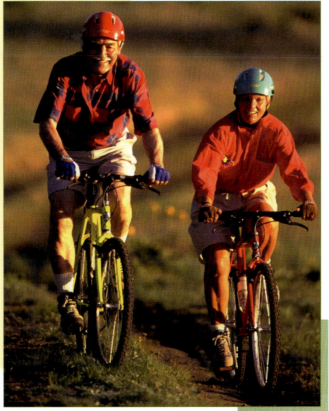

© Brian Drake/SportsChrome

In This Chapter

❏ Explore places to be active—your home, community resources, fitness centers.

❏ Select fitness equipment for your home.

❏ Decide if a personal trainer would be helpful.

❏ Evaluate fitness products and services.

Being physically active can be exciting and energizing. We realize, however, that some people find physical activity unpleasant or boring. In fact, these are among the top 10 reasons that people give for not being active. Certainly, doing the same thing every day in the same place could be boring. But it doesn't have to be that way! When we think of the many types of activities and the variety of places to be active, the possibilities are endless. This chapter is loaded with ways to help you start putting the finishing touches on your fitness program. Everyone must figure out for himself or herself what works and what doesn't. A wealth of resources is out there. You just have to find the right combination for you.

Fortunately, you can be active in lots of places. If you prefer lifestyle physical activity over structured exercise, you have many choices. You can do lifestyle physical activity almost anyplace and anytime. An advantage of lifestyle activity is that you can do tasks and chores that you need and want to do while also working in some activity. And you don't have to change clothes or leave home if you don't want to.

People who enjoy a structured exercise program often prefer going to a fitness center. Today, many fitness centers have classes and membership programs especially for older adults. Other advantages include the opportunity to exercise with others, the variety of equipment available, and staff to assist, supervise, and motivate. You know that if you were to have an emergency, help would be available immediately.

Your decision about where to do structured exercise depends on your personality and individual preferences, as well as practical matters. How far are you willing to drive? What can you afford to spend? Do you want to exercise alone or with others? What time of day works best for you? You should choose the setting for your exercise program carefully because you are much more likely to stay with or expand your routine if the place where you exercise is comfortable, convenient, and suits all your needs.

Be Active at Home

Your home can be an excellent setting in which to establish unshakable physical activity habits. Use action box 7.1 to help you decide if being active at home is right for you.

Action Box 7.1: Should You Be Active at Home?

Mark the advantages and disadvantages of being active at home that apply to you. Add other ideas in the spaces provided.

Advantages	Disadvantages
_____ Saving time by not having to travel to another location	_____ Being distracted by household tasks requiring attention
_____ Enjoying activity in the privacy, safety, and comfort of your home	_____ Being interrupted by family members
_____ Saving money on membership fees	_____ Not having technical advice
_____ Not having to pack a workout bag	_____ Not having supervision or help in case of an emergency
_____ Wearing whatever you want, even your underwear	_____ Not having large fitness equipment to use
_____ Being active while doing the laundry, supervising a child at play, or visiting with your spouse or a companion	_____ Not having the social interaction and motivation of exercising with others
_____ Being a positive role model for your family	_____ Having to buy small fitness equipment
_____ Using your own shower when you are done	List other disadvantages that are important to you here:
_____ Fitting in a workout when it is most convenient for you	
List other advantages that are important to you here:	
_____	_____
_____	_____

Did you mark more advantages than disadvantages? If so, then doing physical activity at home might be right for you. If you marked more disadvantages than advantages, you might find a fitness center or place in your community appealing.

Do You Know?

People age 50 and older who report doing regular activity say that they are active in the following places:

At home	68%	Community center	3%
At work	12%	Somewhere else	10%
Health club	7%		

Those doing moderate activity at home say that they do the following activities:

Walking	54%	Push-ups and stretching	14%
Household chores	35%	Weights	13%
Gardening	18%	Treadmill	10%
Other yard work	17%	Cycling	10%

Data from AARP 2002.

Whether you choose to be active indoors or outdoors at home is usually a matter of environmental conditions and personal preference. If you think that you might prefer indoor activity, ask yourself these questions:

- Is there adequate space to move about freely?

- Do you have the fitness equipment you need for a good workout? See the list of small equipment on the next page.

- Will responsibilities at home—chores, children, telephone calls, or job-related work—distract you?

If you think that you might prefer outdoor activity, be sure to consider these points:

- Do you have a safe, convenient place that is close to your home, such as a quiet street with good sidewalks, a park, school track, or community pathway?

- Is climate, pollen, or air quality an obstacle to year-round outside activity?

- If climate or weather is an obstacle, can you find another place or type of physical activity?

Fortunately, you don't have to limit yourself when you are active at home. You can walk outdoors on weekends or in the early morning when the weather permits. When the weather is bad or you want a change, you can be active indoors with a video or small fitness equipment.

You can now buy high-quality, affordable fitness equipment for your home. Home fitness equipment can add variety and provide a more balanced fitness program. If you are just starting to increase your physical activity, you may be thinking about buying a large piece of equipment, such as a treadmill or stationary cycle. We advise against it at this time. After you have been active for a few months and know more about what is likely to work for you, you'll be in a better position to make a decision about such a major investment.

Small Equipment

If you are interested in equipment, start with something small and less costly. You can use many types of small equipment to enhance your home fitness program. Most of the equipment in the following list is available new for less than US$50. You may want to look for used fitness equipment at garage sales. You can afford to spend a little money on small equipment because you are saving the cost of a fitness center membership. Also, you can create some pieces from items that you have around the house. Try some of these pieces of inexpensive fitness equipment:

Audios—If you listen to music while you exercise, you are likely to enjoy it more and do it longer. Select music that energizes you. Although perhaps not as motivational as music, books on tape provide enjoyment to some people while they walk or cycle. Avoid wearing earphones while walking or jogging outdoors, however, because you may be unable to hear noises that could warn you of potential dangers.

Videos—A variety of high-quality fitness videos are available for rental and purchase. Ask friends to recommend their favorite videos or borrow one to try before you buy. Select a video that is appropriate for your fitness level. Also, check that the instructor leading the session is certified by a recognized institution such as the American Council on Exercise, American College of Sports Medicine, or the Cooper Institute.

Exercise mat—A mat makes floor exercises more comfortable. Vinyl and fabric mats are available. An advantage of a fabric mat is that it is washable. Vinyl mats should be cleaned with a disinfectant frequently. A quilt, bedspread, or large towel can also serve as an exercise mat.

Step counter (pedometer)—This small, inexpensive piece of equipment is one of the best purchases you can make. Step counters are a useful way to monitor your physical activity. Attach your pedometer when you get up in the morning and wear it throughout the day. See chapter 4 for information on buying and using step counters.

Steps—Steps or benches are available for purchase. Start with a step height of 6 inches (15 centimeters) and increase the height as your fitness level improves. Steps probably shouldn't be more than 12 inches (30 centimeters) high. Obtain a video illustrating a stepping program to learn the moves for a good routine.

Heart rate monitors—If you want to know the precise intensity of your activity, a heart rate monitor may help. Typically, a heart rate monitor counts your heart rate (beats per minute) by using electrodes placed against your skin and held in place by a strap around your chest. Some heart rate monitors can be programmed to let you know when you are outside your training zone—whether you are working too hard and should slow down or whether you could work a bit harder, if desired. (Chapter 9 provides more information about the training zone.) Heart rate monitors suitable for beginning walking programs cost as little as US$30. Monitors with more complex features can cost much more. Heart rate monitors are available at most sporting-goods stores or from Web sites.

Hand weights—Small handheld weights (sometimes called dumbbells) come in a variety of styles and sizes. If you are buying dumbbells, select those with grips that are comfortable for you. Choose weights of several sizes, such as 1, 3, 5, 8, and 10 pounds, or 0.5, 1, 3, and 5 kilograms.

You can also create handheld weights from objects around your home. Fill old purses that have handles with heavy objects such as rocks or fill plastic jugs with water or sand. Even cans of food from your pantry can serve as weights. Exercises using handheld weights are discussed in chapter 10.

Strap-on weights—If gripping a dumbbell is difficult for you because of arthritis or other problems, consider weights that strap on your wrists with Velcro. Weights that strap around your ankles are also available, but check with your doctor before using them. Ankle weights of more than 2.5 pounds (1.2 kilograms) are not recommended.

Resistance rubber bands—Resistance bands are available in most sports stores. They take up hardly any space. You can throw them in your suitcase when you travel and take your workout with you. The amount of resistance varies according to the thickness of the band. Bands are typically color coded to indicate the resistance. You can exercise with one band only or use them in combination for greater resistance. Begin with the thinnest band and progress to thicker bands as your strength increases. Chapter 10 discusses exercises using rubber bands.

Fitness ball—These large inflatable plastic balls were first used in rehabilitation programs to help people regain their balance and strength after an injury or surgery. Today, people can do a variety of exercises using a fitness ball.

Large Equipment

After you have some experience with regular physical activity, you may want to consider buying a large piece of fitness equipment for your home. You will need to take some time to select the particular piece of equipment that fits your needs. Then, of course, you must use it regularly and correctly to benefit from your investment.

Using a machine for a few minutes in a store is not a sufficient trial to make an informed decision. Before

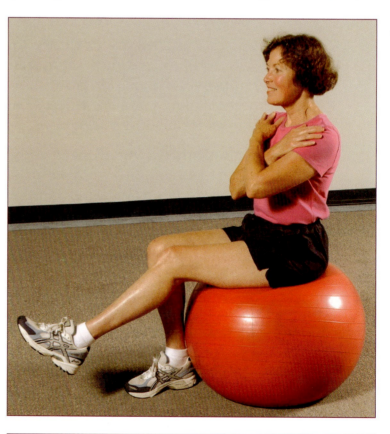

You can use a fitness ball to strengthen the muscles in the trunk of the body.

you buy, obtain access to a machine similar to one that you are considering, perhaps at a fitness center or a YMCA. Ask a fitness instructor to demonstrate correct form and answer your questions. Trying the equipment yourself will ensure that you don't make a big investment that you discover too late does not meet your needs.

If you are considering buying fitness equipment for your home, shop carefully to get the most value for your dollar. Read *Consumer Reports* or visit www.consumerreports.org to get an objective review of a variety of models. Home fitness equipment can be expensive, and, as with most products, a wide range of features and levels of quality is available. You may be able to save money by buying a piece of used fitness equipment. Used equipment, however, may be flawed. Some stores specialize in selling used equipment and offer warranties. Compare the cost of new and used equipment. You may be better off to spend more for something new.

Use the worksheet in action box 7.2 to compare the features of three different models of fitness equipment.

Action Box 7.2: Large Fitness Equipment Checklist

Answer yes or no to each question for each piece of equipment.

Question	Equipment A	Equipment B	Equipment C
Does the manufacturer provide strong customer support (toll-free number or Web site)?			
Does the equipment come with at least a one-year warranty? Does the warranty cover replacement parts? For how long?			
Is electricity required for operation, and does the voltage match your country's electricity (110-120 or 220-240 volt)?			
Does the equipment appear sturdy? Ask about life expectancy.			
Is the cost of the equipment within your budget? More money usually buys better equipment.			
Is the equipment adjustable so that people of different sizes and fitness levels can use it? Adaptability is especially important if several family members want to use the equipment.			

(continued)

➠**Action Box 7.2: Large Fitness Equipment Checklist** *(continued)*

Question	Equipment A	Equipment B	Equipment C
Are training instructions, materials, and videos provided? Are the instructions easy to understand and follow?			
Is the equipment safe and easy to operate? Be sure to try it yourself.			
Can the equipment fit into the space that you have available?			
Is the equipment easy to move and store?			
Does the equipment come assembled, or is it easy to assemble?			
Is the equipment noisy to operate?			
Add other questions here:			

Places to Be Active in Your Community

Your community is likely to have safe outdoor areas and facilities where you can be physically active. Check your local newspaper, city directory, or the Internet for information. Use action box 7.3 to investigate recreational and physical activity resources in your area. Many groups welcome newcomers and provide programs for novices to learn new skills. Start by considering activities that you know you can do or that you've done in the past.

Action Box 7.3: Identify Community Resources for Physical Activity

Use this worksheet to identify the names and locations of fitness resources in your community. Circle the community resource that you think you might like to try in the next couple of weeks. Make a note on your calendar to check it out.

Locations	Notes
Fitness or wellness centers	
Schools, colleges, and universities	
Clubs or leagues	
Parks or recreation centers	
Others	

Personal Profile

Ethel, Age 72

Ethel has just begun to think about becoming more physically active. She lost her husband last year and wants to find a way to make new friends. Ethel asked her son to look on the Internet for local walking programs. He found that a senior walking club meets at a shopping mall during the winter. Here's how Ethel filled out the part of the action box on community resources:

Clubs or leagues *Senior Walking Club—Multi-Plaza Mall* *Call 506-362-4752*	*Mall opens at 7:00 a.m. Enter on Second Avenue. Over 200 members, but less than 20 are walking at any time. There's a registration fee that includes T-shirt and walking kit. Sponsored by Memorial Hospital. Free blood pressure checks monthly. Some walkers go to a coffee shop in the mall after walking.*

Although she was nervous, Ethel took the first step and called the phone number that was listed on the Internet for the walking club. A kind woman named Patricia answered the phone. She told Ethel all the details and invited her to walk with them the next day. Now Ethel walks three days a week with the group at the mall. She has enjoyed meeting new people and becoming more physically active again. The walking club has been a great way to fend off the winter blues.

Fitness Centers

If you think that you might enjoy exercising at a fitness center, you can choose from a large number of well-equipped facilities. Use action box 7.4 to help you decide whether exercising at a fitness center is right for you.

Action Box 7.4: Should You Exercise at a Fitness Center?

Mark the advantages and disadvantages of exercising at a fitness center that apply to you. Add other ideas in the spaces provided.

Did you mark more advantages than disadvantages to using a fitness center? If so, commit to a time this week when you will set an appointment to visit a fitness center near you. See action box 7.5 for questions to ask when you call or visit.

Advantages	Disadvantages
_____ Interacting and socializing with others	_____ Traveling to another location
_____ Getting motivated by exercising with others	_____ Finding a parking space
_____ Having workouts supervised by fitness professionals	_____ Paying fees
_____ Having emergency care readily available in case of injury	_____ Signing a contract
_____ Using a wide range of equipment	_____ Having to pay regardless of use
_____ Having expert advice from staff and trainers	_____ Crowding at popular times
_____ Participating in educational programs	List other disadvantages that are important to you here:
_____ Having screenings and assessments	
_____ Using locker rooms with grooming amenities	
List other advantages that are important to you here:	

If you decide that you are interested in exercising at a fitness center, plan to evaluate several facilities before making a decision. Begin by making a few phone calls. Ask about the following:

- Fees (read-through of contract and waivers, checking of fees against published price list)

- Brochures and applications

- Current membership and capacity

- Special programs or services for older adults

- Training of staff to work with special needs of older people

- Certification of staff by national organizations, such as the American Council on Exercise, American College of Sports Medicine, or the Cooper Institute

- An appointment to speak with a staff member and look at the facility

Select no more than three facilities to visit initially. Schedule your visit at the time of day when you would use the facility, especially if your preferred time is during a peak period, such as after work. Don't be pressured to decide on the spot. Some businesses insist that you sign a contract immediately to get a special discounted price. Be suspicious of high-pressure marketing strategies. Reputable businesses do not use them. Use action box 7.5 as a guide during your evaluation.

Action Box 7.5: Checklist for Evaluating Fitness Facilities

Answer yes or no to each question for each facility.

Question	Facility A	Facility B	Facility C
Convenience. Is the facility convenient? Is it near home or work?			
Hours. Do the hours of operation fit your needs?			
Parking. Is the parking adequate?			
Facilities and equipment. Does the club have the facilities (pool, racquetball courts, aerobics studio) or equipment (free weights, weight machines, cardio machines) that you want to use?			

(continued)

Question	Facility A	Facility B	Facility C
Space. Is the space ample in the showers, locker rooms, and fitness rooms, and on the courts and tracks?			
Availability. Is space and equipment available at the time when you would visit?			
Physical condition. Are the facility and equipment clean, neat, well maintained, and in good working order?			
Air quality. Are the temperature, humidity, and ventilation controlled and comfortable at peak times?			
Programs. Does the facility provide comprehensive fitness programming (cardiovascular, strength, and flexibility training) as well as sports activities? Is special programming offered for older adults?			
Special services. Does the facility provide comprehensive health and fitness services (fitness assessments, goals and action plans, physical therapy, arthritis therapy, cardiac rehabilitation, weight loss programs, nutrition counseling)?			
Staff. Are staff experienced, well qualified, and certified by recognized agencies like the American Red Cross (CPR and first aid), the American College of Sports Medicine (ACSM), the American Council on Exercise, and the Cooper Institute? Are staff healthy role models? Are they friendly and supportive? Are personal trainers available?			
Supportive systems. Are activities available to encourage adherence (recognition programs, challenges and contests, monitoring systems, recreational leagues)?			
Safety and security. Are safety and security practices emphasized (written policies and procedures, appropriate signage)?			
Cost. Is the membership fee affordable for you? Are there any hidden costs? Must you sign a contract?			
Add other considerations here:			

Personal Trainers

Some people hire personal trainers to help them with their fitness programs. A personal trainer will design and supervise an individualized program that will monitor your progress and help you master skills and get results. A trainer may perform one-on-one training sessions in your home or at a fitness center. Fees range from US$25 to US$100 per session, depending on the length of the session, location, and the trainer's experience and credentials. You may get a better value by buying a package of sessions rather than single sessions. Some fitness centers include a few personal training sessions with staff as part of services for new members.

Although working with a personal trainer has advantages, there are potential disadvantages as well. Besides being expensive, sessions may cause clients to become dependent on their trainers. Some people exercise only when they are with their trainers. If they discontinue their sessions with their trainers for some reason, they are likely to give up their exercise.

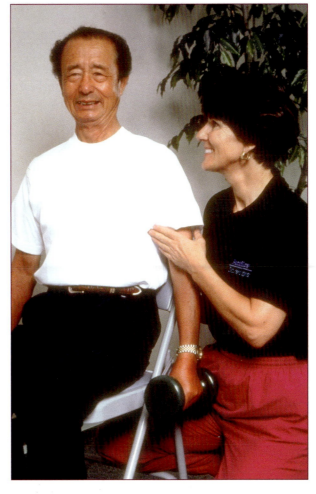

Would you enjoy working with a personal trainer?

Before hiring a personal trainer, ask yourself these questions: How many sessions can I afford? What is the benefit for me? Will I exercise more regularly with a trainer? Will I get better results? Will I be able to stay with the program when I discontinue the sessions?

If you decide to hire a personal trainer, conduct face-to-face interview with several trainers before making a final decision. Use action box 7.6 to conduct your interview and compare the trainers. Add other questions that are important to you at the bottom of the form.

More than likely, your choice will be influenced by whether you like the trainer and think that you would enjoy working with him or her. Make sure that you hire someone who is qualified and will help you get the most from your fitness program. Have a trial session before making a final decision.

Action Box 7.6: Questions for Personal Trainers

Question	Trainer A	Trainer B	Trainer C
What certifications do you have? Ask the trainer to show proof, including first aid and CPR certification. If a personal trainer has no certification and is not trained in CPR, do not hire the trainer.			
How much experience do you have as a personal trainer? Have you worked with people my age (or who have a health problem such as _____)? Ask for a list of previous and current clients.			
Do you have professional liability insurance?			
Do you conduct screenings and fitness assessments before you begin an exercise program with a client?			
What would the program include? Will it include exercises to improve my aerobic fitness, muscle fitness, and balance?			
Will you provide a program for me to follow on my own, between sessions?			
What kind of improvement or upgrade can I expect after a specific time (such as six weeks)?			
When and where would the workouts take place?			
What is your relationship with the health or fitness club (if the session is at a club)?			
What is the cost per session? Must I sign a contract? Can I terminate it at any time? Am I charged if I cancel an appointment?			
What happens if I am injured during a session?			
Write other questions here:			

The Truth About Fitness Products and Services

As you start to shop for various fitness products and services, you will be amazed at what's out there. Unfortunately, not all the products and services that you see and hear about on television and radio or read about in best-selling books or on popular Web sites are reliable. The desire for the quick fix makes people vulnerable to scientifically unsound health and fitness products and services.

Be cautious! Don't believe everything that you read or hear. "Consumer beware" is good advice. To assess the reliability of any health or fitness resource, ask these questions:

■ Who is saying it? What credentials, training, or experience qualifies the person to make the claims? Even people who claim to have advanced educational or medical degrees may provide misleading information. In addition, not all educational and nonprofit institutions are credible. Celebrities with no specific training or expertise in a given field often endorse worthless products. They are probably receiving generous compensation for promoting products. Beware of paid endorsements.

■ Does what is being claimed seem too good to be true? Does it promise to be quick and easy? If it sounds too good to be true, it probably is!

■ Where are the claims being said? Some media are more careful than others in checking their sources before publishing information. You can trust peer-reviewed scientific journals, but most people don't read these publications. Scientific sources are frequently quoted, but research findings are often misinterpreted or taken out of context. "Infomercials" and "advertorials," which are quickly becoming a common source of consumer information, can easily confuse the buyer. Many complex issues are reduced to sound bites that make good copy for the evening news but fail to give an accurate overall picture.

Summary

Congratulations! You are more than half way through *Fitness After 50.* You have covered much of the basics of physical activity: how it is beneficial, what to do if you have special conditions, what you need to get started, how to find time to be active, which types of fitness are most important to older adults, and where to go to be active. As you prepare to develop your fitness plan, could you use a little help from your friends and family? If you think about a goal that you achieved in the past, you probably would say that others were important to your success—a teacher, coach, parent, sibling, or friend. The next chapter helps you think about how you can get support from others.

Chapter Checklist

Following are some ways in which you can apply what you have learned in this chapter to your daily life. Over the next few days and weeks try to do as many of these activities as possible.

❏ If you are just getting started, determine where you would like to do physical activity. If you plan to be active away from home, be sure to find a convenient place. Make plans to call or visit possible places this week.

❏ If you plan to be active at home, consider any small fitness equipment that you might like to use. Don't make a major investment in large equipment until you have been active for a while and are sure that you would use the equipment regularly.

❏ If you are already active, investigate new places in your community where you can be active. For variety, plan to try a new fitness location at least once this month.

❏ If you think you might like to work with a personal trainer, get names of trainers from a fitness center and schedule interviews. You might also ask friends who have worked with trainers to give you a recommendation. Have a trial session before making a final decision.

Word Search

See if you can find 10 important words from this chapter in the grid that follows. Words appear forward and backward in rows, columns, and diagonals. The solution is shown on page 232.

```
Y T E F A S H J I N E O O N T
S D D W P Y M F E C N U S O Q
R E Q U I P M E N T X T O I B
E E K L M X R E G H M D U T G
Z M T H Y B I G B F U O D A K
G Q O N A N B S Y E A O E C C
D W R H E W R E G V Q R P I T
T X C V X C Q N L O N S V F B
V H N C U L S P D L C J N I K
I O W J Y T S S Z Y S N N T K
C V X M A U U P E X W D R R Y
R E N I A R T L A N O S R E P
Z J G C A A H J J O T W J C P
T T V C N S G Y R Y A I U F X
D X X T Y P U S N O K R F E Y
```

Certification   Fitness center   Outdoors
Convenience   Home   Personal trainer
Dumbbells   Indoors   Safety
Equipment

Get a Little Help From Your Friends

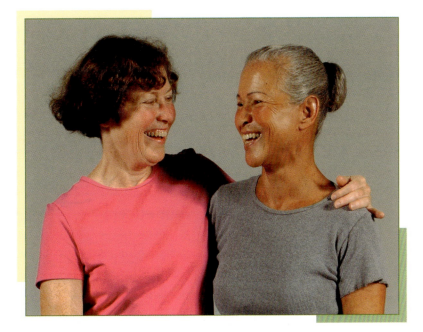

In This Chapter

❏ Plan to involve others in your activity program.

❏ Practice assertive communication when making plans to be active.

❏ Think of ways to make physical activity fun.

People need social support to attain and maintain habits, including regular physical activity, especially when getting started. This chapter suggests ways in which you can involve others in your physical activity program. You may want an activity partner or choose to join a group class, or you may just need someone to help with household chores while you go out for a walk. Regardless of whether you are part of a group or alone, physical activity should and can be a lot of fun. Your physical activity should be a highlight of your day.

Involve Others

Consider whether you would enjoy doing physical activity with another person or with a group. Many people report that joining others for physical activity makes it more fun and helps them stick with it. Having someone remind you to be active or let you know that you were missed if you skip a session can be motivating. Some people say that they are more likely to show up for a session if they know that someone else depends on them to be there. Use the tips in this chapter to help you get the support that you need to stay active.

Having an activity partner or being part of a class or team can help you stay motivated to stay active. But to fit physical activity into your life, you may need support in other areas as well. Here are some ways that a partner, spouse, family member, or friend might help you stay active:

- Assume tasks or chores so that you have time to be active
- Ask how you are doing and praise your efforts
- Remind you to be active
- Share in a reward when you achieve a goal
- Challenge you when you lapse

Personal Profile

Susan, Age 58

Susan had walked with her friend Karen for more than five years. They met at a corner in their neighborhood every morning at 6:30 a.m. and walked for about 45 minutes. Susan moved to another city because of a new job. Several months after the move, Susan was having difficulty staying with her morning physical activity program. She had not realized how important having a partner was to her activity plan. From time to time, Susan saw a woman from down the street walking, but not at a regular time. She decided to ask the woman if they could walk together at a set time each morning. The neighbor agreed. Susan sent Karen an e-mail to tell her that she was getting back on track. She asked Karen to send her a weekly e-mail reminder to ask about how she is doing.

Rob, Age 72, and Evelyn, Age 73

Rob and Evelyn, both single, first met on a walking–jogging trail in a city park on a crisp autumn morning. Neither can remember exactly how their conversation began, but they enjoyed talking for nearly 30 minutes as they continued to walk. When Evelyn completed the distance that was her typical program, Rob asked if she would like to go to brunch at a nearby restaurant. Normally, Evelyn would not have accepted an invitation from a stranger, but she felt safe because she would be driving her own car and eating in a public place. They enjoyed brunch and made a date for dinner later in the week (again Evelyn drove her own car). Their friendship progressed slowly over several months as they found that they had many common interests besides physical activity. Today Evelyn and Rob are married. They enjoy telling others that a benefit of an activity program is finding a mate!

Evaluate Your Support System

Consider who could support your physical activity program. You'll probably find it easiest to think about involving people close to you—family members, neighbors, and coworkers. You can also use physical activity as a way to make new friends. You will meet some kind and interesting people while engaged in physical activity or recreational fitness activities. What types of support do you need and want? Use action box 8.1 to identify people around you who can support your activity program.

Action Box 8.1: Who Can Help?

Write the names of one or two people who could give you each type of support listed here. Leave areas blank if you do not need or want that type of support. Choose one type of support to seek this week. Start thinking about how you will approach people who can provide that type of support.

I will seek the following type of support this week:

Type of support	Who can help?
Emotional challenge—people who challenge you to attain your goals	
Listening support—people who listen to your concerns and problems without judging	

(continued)

Type of support	Who can help?
Feedback and appraisal—people who tell you how you're doing and praise your efforts and progress	
Role models and partners—people who share similar experiences, values, and views related to physical activity	
Experts and information support—people who know more about physical activity than you do and whose advice you can trust	
Add other types of help or support that you want here:	

If after evaluating your support system you find that you are lacking a specific type of support that you need, try to build support in that area. If you can't list more than one name for each type of support, you might consider ways to increase the depth of your support system in that area. Here are a few tips for adding to your support system:

- Join organizations, clubs, or religious groups and become involved.

- Let others get to know the real you. Be willing to share personal experiences.

- Question others to learn about their interests and needs rather than talk about yourself.

- Be a taker as well as a giver. Look for mutually supportive relationships.

- Learn to ask for the type of support that you need and want. Be specific when you ask for support. Don't wait for others to read your mind. Tell them what would and would not be helpful.

- Know that some people may not accept or adjust to your new lifestyle. Be prepared to modify old relationships, at least for a while, if someone sabotages your efforts to be active.

- Actively avoid the naysayers who put down or diminish your efforts to be active in any way.

- Seek out people with similar values and habits who can be supportive. If you are just starting to be active, identify a good role model. Ask how he or she succeeded in staying active. Try to picture yourself as an active person.

- Don't be afraid to set limits when the actions of other people might interfere with your plans to be active. Follow these three steps to establish boundaries:
    - Describe the specific behavior that is bothering you and how you're feeling.
    - Specify the action that you'd like the person to change.
    - Tell the person what will happen if he or she is able or not able to do what you have requested.

Personal Profile

Jeff, Age 67

Jeff decided to become involved in a physical activity program after his doctor told him that being active would help him control his blood pressure. He found a fitness center that provides special membership fees and programs for retired people who use the facility between two and four o'clock in the afternoons. Unfortunately, that was the time when he usually played cards with the guys. When Jeff asked the group if they could move the game of hearts to the evening so that he could exercise, they gave him a hard time. Although he explained that he was exercising for his health, they still tried to talk him out of going. "You're fine," they said. "You're healthy as a horse! You don't need to waste your time or money at a gym." Jeff assertively stuck with his plan to be active, and the group agreed to reschedule the game so that he could play. The negative comments about his physical activity became less frequent over time. Jeff's friends noticed that he seemed to be feeling better. He reported that his blood pressure had come down enough that his doctor stopped his medicine. After several invitations to the group to be his guest at the fitness center, Bill took Jeff up on his offer. Soon, Bill joined the fitness center, and Jeff helped him get started with physical activity. Now it's two against two when the topic of physical activity comes up during a card game.

Learn to Communicate Assertively

The first step in building support is to know the types of support that you need and want and who might provide it. Then you must make your wants and needs known in a specific and assertive way. Learning to communicate assertively and directly can help you stay active when people or situations block the way to your goals.

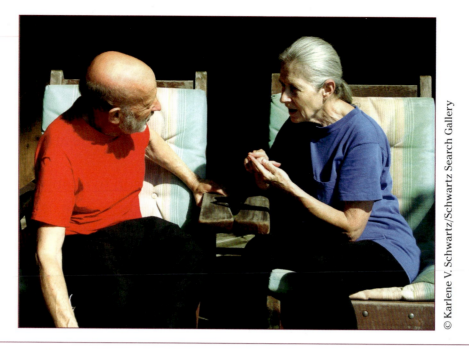

© Karlene V. Schwartz/Schwartz Search Gallery

You are more likely to get results with assertive communication, which is calm and direct.

Nonassertive and aggressive styles are both indirect forms of communication. People with an aggressive style might overreact and lose their temper. Called hot reactors, they may be at greater risk for coronary heart disease and other stress-related illnesses. People with a nonassertive communication style may withdraw and use the silent treatment. But people with an assertive style of communication are calm and direct. They take time to think before responding. Instead of using a "You" statement, an assertive person uses an "I" statement.

More tips for assertive communication appear in the following list. Almost everyone can benefit by trying to communicate more assertively. Try to apply the tips to your daily life. Complete action box 8.2 to practice how you would respond in situations related to your physical activity plans.

Tips for Assertive Communication

- Speak firmly and make eye contact.
- Avoid hints and sarcasm.
- Use your voice and body language to communicate confidence.
- Remain calm and don't let your emotions interfere.
- Take time to think over your response. If necessary, indicate a specific time when you can respond so it doesn't appear that you're avoiding the issue.
- Plan and practice what you will say so that you will feel prepared and confident to deal with the situation.

Action Box 8.2:   How Would You Respond?

Write assertive responses to these comments or actions by others.

Situation: Jo has bought a colorful, tight-fitting new outfit for her group fitness class. She's on her way to the community center for the class when she sees her friend Margie.

Comment: Margie says, "What are you trying to prove by wearing those exercise clothes?"

Assertive response:

Situation: David is still jogging, although slower, at age 70. His friend Randall has always been inactive.

Comment: Randall says, "Why don't you slow down and act your age? You know, you're not so young!"

Assertive response:

If You Must Say No

When you choose physical activity over inactivity, you must at times say no to requests. At these times, learn to negotiate. Consider the other person's requests but don't give up on your plan to be active. Be direct instead of making excuses. Here are some ways to be assertive when someone asks you to change your physical activity plans.

Instead of saying, "You're always planning things that interfere with my activity time," say, "Part of me would like to go to the movie with you, but the other part is saying that I really need to be active."

Instead of saying, "Your request to come in early every day is unreasonable," say, "I don't want to give up my morning workout to meet early every day this week. But I can come in early two days and stay late two days."

If You Need to Ask for Help

Sometimes you will need to request help from others so that you can be active. Part of taking care of yourself is asking for help when you need it. Most people are happy to help if the request gives them a choice to say yes or no. Also, try to consider the other person's needs and feelings.

When making requests, give clear, specific information that will help others decide whether to say yes or no. For example, say the following:

"Would you consider a vacation this year that includes ways to be physically activity? Think about it, and we'll talk more later."

"Would you like to participate in the Fun Run in two weeks? It's OK if you say no."

Start to think about requests that you may need to make related to your physical activity program. Complete action box 8.3.

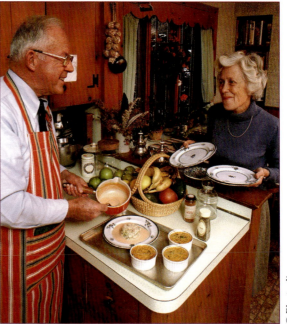

© Photodisc

Ask someone to help you with a household chore so that you can make time for physical activity.

Action Box 8.3: How Will You Make Requests?

What requests might you need to make to gain support for your physical activity? Look back at your responses in action box 8.1: Who Can Help? on pages 131 and 132. Whom will you ask? Write your requests in the following space.

Whom I will ask:	What I will say:

Which of these requests are you ready to make this week? Circle the request and make plans to talk with that person.

Make Physical Activity Enjoyable

Regardless of the type of activity you do and whether you do it with a group, partner, personal trainer, or alone, you aren't likely to stay with physical activity long term if you don't enjoy it. You won't do what you don't like. You can make your physical activity enjoyable by adding some humor and fun. As you learned in chapter 5, rewards are another way to make physical activity fun.

We have never heard anyone say that he or she gave up physical activity because it was too much fun. Here are a few ways in which others have added fun and humor to their physical activity routines. Circle the ones that you'd enjoy doing.

1. Tell jokes with your partner.
2. March along while you call out chants as a military drill sergeant would.
3. Wear unmatched or bright-colored clothing or a funny hat.
4. Race your partner to the next landmark.
5. Tie bells to your shoelaces.
6. Put a flag on your bicycle.
7. Play I Spy with your partner while walking in the neighborhood.
8. Say hello in a foreign language to everyone you see.
9. Enter a running or walking event and wear a costume.
10. Participate in an event to raise money for a charity.

What other ideas do you have for making physical activity fun? Try one this week.

Summary

This chapter has introduced two important skills to help you become and stay active: involving others and communicating assertively. Building support for your activity is critical, especially if you are just getting started. Having support is also important if you are challenging yourself to try something new or reach a new level. The social aspects of physical activity also make it fun. Activity is one of the best ways to enjoy relationships or make new friends. In the next chapter, we'll finish your plan for aerobic fitness.

Chapter Checklist

Following are some ways in which you can apply what you have learned in this chapter to your daily life. Over the next few days and weeks try to do as many of these activities as possible.

❑ Think of at least one way in which you can involve someone else in your physical activity program. Don't expect others to read your mind. Ask today in an assertive way.

❏   Focus on making physical activity fun. Do at least one thing each week to add some fun to your physical activity.

❏   Continue to practice affirmations regularly. Think of affirmations as intangible rewards for being active.

❏   Review your list of pros (advantages) and cons (disadvantages) for being physically active. Have you been able to eliminate some barriers to being active? Is your list of pros becoming longer? When you see more pros than cons for physical activity, you are well on your way to making activity a regular habit.

Word Search

See if you can find 10 important words from this chapter in the grid that follows. Words appear forward and backward in rows, columns, and diagonals. The solution is shown on page 232.

```
Z S X M S F T A P R Q P E Y J
U Q O J K X E G T Q H L S A Z
Q O Q C O E G G V H Y G S N V
E E L B I P L R F T Y S D R F
X Z M E A A U E S U E U A E I
L F H E L P L S D R N F C N Q
L C Q O E U H S T O R A C T E
W H V L X W G I U V M Z Y R F
R O S S C T V V X P U E F A Z
Z Q N R F E C E Y D P R L P K
E G N E L L A H C B W O O O H
O U P R B L L V T F V X R E R
C O M M U N I C A T I O N T J
L C S J K H Y R C X O Q V A J
X I W V U C J F G B A B N C N
```

Aggressive   Fun   Role model
Assertive   Help   Social support
Challenge   Partner   Style
Communication

Create Your Aerobic Fitness Program

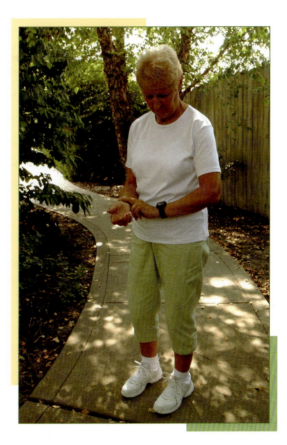

In This Chapter

❏ Learn about the FITT plan for fitness.

❏ Learn ways to know how hard you are exercising.

❏ Use our model aerobic fitness program to develop one of your own.

Perhaps you have found ways to be active through your lifestyle and now you'd like to explore structured exercise. In chapter 6 you explored several of the types of aerobic fitness programs that are popular with people over 50—walking, water activities, and stationary cycling and other cardio machines. Have you found one that appeals to you?

These types of exercise are more structured than lifestyle physical activity. Sometimes structured exercise is more intense than lifestyle physical activity, but it doesn't have to be. Structured exercise, however, does require planning and organizing. The tools in this chapter will help you develop a plan that will work for you. Follow our step-by-step approach and you'll be on your way.

In the early 1970s scientists came up with a simple way to help people plan effective physical activity programs. You may have heard of the FITT plan:

F = Frequency

I = Intensity

T = Time

T = Type

The FITT plan works for both lifestyle physical activity and structured exercise programs. See table 9.1 for a simple comparison of lifestyle physical activity and a structured aerobic fitness program. The biggest difference between the two is that for structured exercise you are setting aside a specific time of day to be physically active.

You can also use the FITT plan to design all types of structured exercise programs, not just programs for aerobic fitness. In the remainder of

Table 9.1 Lifestyle Physical Activity Versus Structured Aerobic Fitness Program

FITT aspect	Lifestyle physical activity	Structured aerobic fitness
Frequency	Every day or nearly every day	Minimum of three days per week for vigorous activity and five days per week for moderate activity
Intensity	Moderate intensity, equivalent to brisk walking	Moderate to vigorous intensity
Time	Minimum of 30 minutes over the course of the day	Minimum of 20 minutes per session for vigorous activity and 30 minutes per session for moderate activity
Type	Activities of daily living that get you up and moving, such as climbing stairs, vacuuming, or gardening	Exercises that use the large muscle groups, such as walking, jogging, sports, and bicycling

this chapter we will focus on planning for aerobic fitness. Chapter 10 will provide exercise programs to improve your muscle strength and endurance, joint flexibility, and balance. Even if you're not quite ready to plan an entire physical activity program, this chapter will help you think more about physical activity. Building knowledge is important in the early stages of change. You may find that you're not ready for a full-blown workout but that you like the ideas given for warming up and cooling down. Take any ideas that you learn from this chapter and make them your own!

How Often?

Frequency (F) is the number of times that you exercise each week. Depending on the intensity you choose, you should perform aerobic exercise three to five times per week. Fewer days are required if you do higher intensity activities. Of course, you can choose to be active every day of the week. You can do a combination of lifestyle physical activity, structured exercises, and leisure or recreational activities.

How Hard?

Intensity (I) is how hard you are working. Lifestyle physical activity is typically of moderate intensity. Aerobic exercises use primarily the large muscles in the legs and buttocks. However, swimming is also an aerobic activity, and it uses primarily muscles in the arms and shoulders. Your heart must work harder (beat faster) to supply these muscles with the oxygen that they need to work. Aerobic exercise can be of moderate or vigorous intensity. Table 9.2 gives examples of physical activities of moderate and vigorous intensity. Any activity less intense than brisk walking is usually

Table 9.2 Examples of Moderate and Vigorous Physical Activities for People Over Age 50

Moderate-intensity activities	Vigorous-intensity activities
If you have been inactive for a long time, you will need to work up to these activities gradually:	If you have been inactive for a long time or have some of the conditions discussed in chapter 3, do not start with these activities:
Walking briskly	
Swimming or water activities	Climbing stairs or hills
Stationary cycling	Jogging
Gardening (mowing, raking)	Swimming laps
Mopping floors	Digging holes
Golf (without a cart)	Shoveling snow
Doubles tennis	Cross-country skiing
Rowing	Downhill skiing
Dancing	Singles tennis

considered low intensity. Although new findings have shown that exercise intensity doesn't have to be vigorous to offer benefits, you should do moderate-intensity activities to gain significant health benefits.

You can use several methods to know whether you are exercising at the right intensity—hard enough to benefit your health but not so hard that exercising is not safe. You can compare your pulse to your training zone, assess your level of perceived exertion, or do a talk test.

Check Your Pulse

Follow the directions in action box 9.1 to take your pulse rate while exercising. Then check to see whether your pulse rate is within your training zone (a heart rate range that is calculated for you). The training zone will not work for you if your pulse rate is likely to be inaccurate for any reason, such as taking a medicine that affects your heart rate. If your pulse rate is below the lower number of your training zone, you would probably benefit by picking up the pace a bit. Having a pulse rate above the training zone is not necessarily a problem. You simply may be a person with a higher than average maximal heart rate. If your pulse rate is above the training zone and you feel fine and are not gasping for breath, there is no major need to slow down.

Action Box 9.1: Taking Your Pulse During Exercise

These instructions will help you take your pulse and calculate your training zone.

How to Take Your Pulse

You'll need a watch or clock with a second hand or digital indicator. Take your pulse immediately after you stop exercising. If you wait too long, your pulse rate will begin to decline. To locate your pulse, place the first two fingers (never the thumb) of one hand on the inside of your wrist near the thumb of your other hand. Count the beats for 15 seconds. Multiply your count by four to get the beats per minute. Determine whether your pulse rate is within your training zone.

A more accurate way to take your pulse during activity is to wear a heart rate monitor. See chapter 7 for information about heart rate monitors.

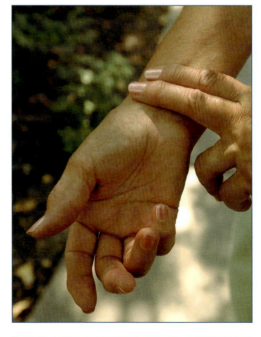

Continue to walk, if possible, while taking your pulse.

How to Find Your Training Zone

Do not use the training-zone method if you

- take medicines (such as beta-blockers) that change your heart rate,
- have a pacemaker,
- have an irregular heart rhythm (called atrial fibrillation),
- have difficulty taking your pulse, or
- have any other condition that affects your pulse rate.

The training zone is defined as 50 to 80 percent of your maximum heart rate. Maximum heart rate is the highest rate that your heart can beat. Exercise that requires your heart to beat faster than the maximum rate is unsafe, and you can't sustain it for long.

Maximum heart rate = 220 minus your age

Training zone = 50 to 80 percent of maximum heart rate

For example, if you are 67 the following numbers apply:

Maximum heart rate = 220 − 67 = 153

$0.5 \times 153 = 77$

$0.8 \times 153 = 122$

Training zone = 77 to 122 beats per minute (bpm)

Use the following chart to find your training zone.

Your age	Your maximum heart rate (bpm)	Your training zone (bpm) 50%	60%	70%	80%
50	170	85	102	119	136
55	165	83	99	116	132
60	160	80	96	112	128
65	155	78	93	109	124
70	150	75	90	105	120
75	145	73	87	102	116
80	140	70	84	98	112
85	135	68	81	95	108
90	130	65	78	91	104
95	125	63	75	88	100
100	120	60	72	84	96

bpm = beats per minute

Rate Your Level of Exertion

An even easier ways that anyone can use to check the intensity of exercise is the Borg rating of perceived exertion (RPE) scale. You use a scale to make a subjective appraisal of how hard you are working. More than 40 years of use has proved the reliability of this scale for measuring exercise intensity. The Borg scale is especially useful if you are taking medicines that alter your pulse rate.

Look at the Borg scale of perceived exertion in table 9.3. The scale has numbers from 6 to 20. To rate your exercise intensity, pick the number that best describes your overall feeling of how hard you are exercising. To do moderate-intensity activity, your aerobic activity should feel "somewhat hard" (between 12 and 14 on the Borg scale). At this level of intensity, on a cold day you should breathe more rapidly and your body should feel comfortably warm. On a warm day, or even at room temperature, you should breathe more rapidly and sweat at least a little.

Table 9.3 Borg Scale of Perceived Exertion

Level	Perceived exertion
6	No exertion at all
7	
	Extremely light
8	
9	Very light
10	
11	Light
12	
13	Somewhat hard
14	
15	Hard (heavy)
16	
17	Very hard
18	
19	Extremely hard
20	Maximal exertion

Physical signs

9 corresponds to "very light" exercise. For a normal, healthy person, it is like walking slowly at his or her own pace for some minutes.

13 on the scale is "somewhat hard" exercise, but it still feels OK to continue.

17 "very hard" is very strenuous. A healthy person can still go on, but he or she really has to push him- or herself. It feels very heavy, and the person is very tired.

19 on the scale is an extremely strenuous exercise level. For most people, this is the most strenuous exercise they have ever experienced.

G. Borg, 1998, *Borg's Perceived Exertion and Pain Scales* (Champaign, IL: Human Kinetics), 47. © Gunnar Borg, 1970, 1985, 1994, 1998.

Do a Talk Test

Another simple way to know how hard you are working is the talk test. This test is particularly easy to use while walking. You should be able to breathe comfortably and deeply at all times during physical activity. If you are exercising with a partner, you should be able to talk. If you are breathing so hard that you can't easily talk, your activity may be too intense. You are probably working too hard and should slow down. On the other hand, if you are so comfortable that you can sing, you could probably work a bit harder.

How Long?

Time (T) means how long each structured exercise session lasts. If you are just starting, your total time could be as short as a few minutes. After a while you should work up to 30 minutes of moderate-intensity exercise. If you are doing vigorous exercise, work up to a minimum of 20 minutes. Regardless of the intensity, try to do structured exercise without stopping. Add time for warm-up and cool-down before and after your exercise session. You can get even greater benefit by increasing your exercise time. (By comparison, if you are adopting the lifestyle approach, your goal is to accumulate a total of 30 minutes of physical activity over the course of the day. Lifestyle bouts of physical activity could be as brief as 10 minutes each.)

Warm-Up and Cool-Down

Most people tend to jump right in to their exercise without doing a proper warm-up. Resist the urge to start too fast by warming up for about five minutes before you do any type of exercise. The purpose of the warm-up is to prepare your joints and muscles for the work that you are about to do. Warming up will also minimize muscle soreness following the exercise. Exercises that increase the heart rate, such as walking, marching in place, or light body weight activities are particularly appropriate. Before you begin a specific type of exercise you should also move the joints through the movements that you will do when you increase your exercise intensity. For example, the best way to warm up for a brisk walk is to walk slowly.

Cooling down is just as important as warming up. Take about five minutes to cool down at the end of your exercise session. Keep moving while you cool down and allow your body to return gradually to a resting state. Continue to perform the same movements as you exercise, but at a slower pace (for example, walk slowly following a brisk walk). Add a few stretches at the end of the cool-down period. You'll usually find that stretching at the end of the workout is easier than it is at the beginning. You should be able to extend the stretch because your muscles are warm. Descriptions of two warm-up (or cool-down) exercises follow. Chapter 10 provides examples of stretching exercises.

Tai Chi Move

Stand tall with your feet shoulder-width apart and your arms at your sides. As you inhale, bring your arms out and up, palms facing toward the ceiling until your hands meet above your head. Begin to exhale as you lower your hands, still pressed together, to the center of your chest. Relax your arms to the starting position. Repeat 10 times, taking one deep breath per move.

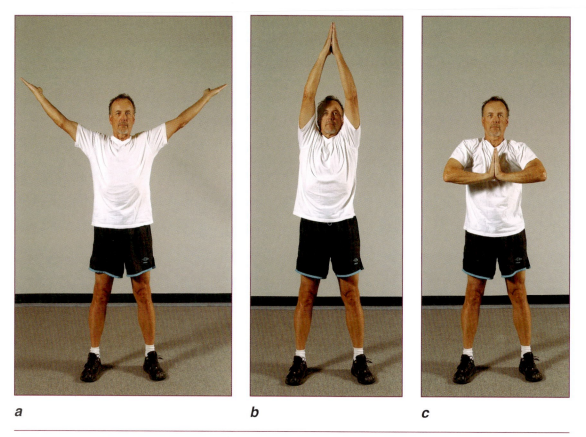

a   *b*   *c*

Tai chi move: *(a)* arms out and up, *(b)* hands meet above head, *(c)* hands together at center of chest.

Side Steps

Stand with your feet together and hold both arms to your right side at shoulder height. Take a wide step sideways with your left foot and smoothly follow with your right foot. At the same time, swing your arms in a circle, beginning on the right and ending on your left. Finish with your arms at your left side, feet together. Repeat in the opposite direction. If warming up, do this move at a brisk clip. If cooling down, do the move slowly.

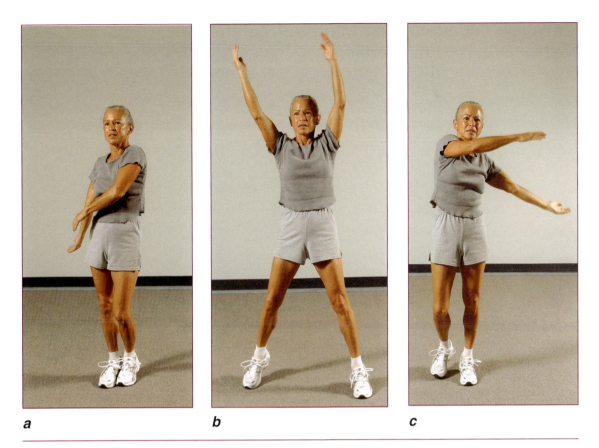

a   *b*   *c*

Side steps: *(a)* both arms to right side, *(b)* wide step sideways while swinging arms in a circle, and *(c)* both arms to left side

Model Aerobic Fitness Program

Our model aerobic fitness program will help you plan a safe, effective routine. The program will also be one that you can stay with because you make adjustments as you go. The model program uses the FITT plan, focused on frequency, intensity, and time. Choose the type of aerobic activity that appeals most to you. The time focus is on minutes of exercise rather than distance covered or pace.

In the next chapter, we'll add strength-building exercises, stretching, and exercises to improve your balance for a total fitness program.

If you are just starting, use our model aerobic exercise plan shown in table 9.4. Choose one type of aerobic activity to focus on for the first few months. We suggest that you try walking, swimming, water aerobics, or stationary cycling. Suppose that you choose walking. From looking at the first row in table 9.4, you can see that in the first week you would plan to walk three or four times (maybe Monday, Wednesday, Friday, and possibly Saturday). After a brief warm-up period, you'd walk for 10 minutes without stopping at a brisk pace, so that your RPE would be around 12 to 14 on the 20-point scale. However, if you find it difficult to walk continuously for 10 minutes, it is fine to walk for a shorter period until you can go for 10

Table 9.4 Model Aerobic Fitness Program (Select One Type of Exercise)

Week	Frequency (times per week)	Intensity*	Time** (minutes per session)
1	3-4	RPE 12-14 (for all weeks)	10
2	4		10
3	4-5		15
4	4-5		20
5	4-5		25
6	5		30
7	5		30
8	5		30-35
9	5		30-35
10	5		30-40
11	5		30-40
12	5		30-45

*Use your training zone, the ratings of perceived exertion, or the talk test to evaluate your exercise intensity.

**Include three to five minutes for warm-up and cool-down at the beginning and end of the exercise session.

minutes without stopping. In the second week, you would follow the same plan but would try to walk on four days.

To develop your own plan, decide which aerobic activity you want to do. Then plan the first few weeks of your program using table 9.4. Keep a record of the exercise that you actually do as you implement your plan. If the program seems too easy as you get started, you can progress to the next week. If the program seems too hard, cut back some or stay at the same level for more than one week. Take it slow at first. You should try to progress to at least week 6 of this model—doing 30 minutes of daily aerobic exercise.

If this is your first time at trying a structured exercise program, you may want to stay with one type of aerobic exercise for a while. Some people wait years before adding another type of aerobic exercise. If you plan to do only one type of aerobic exercise at this time, skip to page 149 and set a goal to implement your aerobic fitness plan.

If you have been doing one type of aerobic exercise for at least 12 weeks, you may want to add another. When you add a different type of exercise, you will need to adjust your program. Table 9.5 shows a model for adding a second type of aerobic exercise. Suppose that you have completed at

Table 9.5 Model Aerobic Fitness Program—Adding a Second Type of Aerobic Exercise

Week	First type frequency (times per week)	First type time* (minutes per session)	Second type frequency (times per week)	Second type time* (minutes per session)	Intensity**
13	4	Minimum of 30 (for all weeks)	1	10	RPE 12-14 (for all weeks)
14	4		1	15	
15	4		1	20	
16	3		2	15	
17	3		2	20	
18	3		2	25	
19	2-3		2-3	30	
20	2-3		2-3	30	
21	2-3		2-3	30	
22	2-3		2-3	30	
23	2-3		2-3	30	
24	2-3		2-3	30	

*Include three to five minutes for warm-up and cool-down at the beginning and end of the exercise session.

**Use your training zone, the rating of perceived exertion, or the talk test to evaluate your exercise intensity.

least 12 weeks of walking, walking five days a week for 30 minutes each session. Now you want to add stationary cycling to your exercise program. In week 13 you should do your regular walking program on four days at 30 minutes per session. You should plan to do stationary cycling on one day during week 13. Because the cycling will feel more intense to you than your walking does, you should cycle for only 10 minutes in that session. Over the next two weeks, add more time to your cycling session. When you can cycle for at least 20 minutes without stopping, you can add another cycling day, but you should cut out a day of walking and cut back on your cycling time as shown in the table.

Set a Realistic Goal

One of the challenges of starting an exercise program to improve your aerobic fitness is setting a realistic goal. Many people make the mistake of expecting too much too soon. They start out working too hard, quickly become discouraged, maybe even get injured, and give up on the program before they see any benefits. Remember from chapter 5 that your goal should be specific, challenging but realistic, written on paper, and tied to a reward. You might also want to share your goal with another person so that you can be accountable to him or her. Complete action box 9.2 to set a goal to implement your aerobic exercise plan.

Action Box 9.2:   My Aerobic Exercise Goal

Question or task	Example	My goal
What do you want to accomplish long term? Be specific.	My goal over six weeks is to be able to walk for 30 minutes at a brisk pace without stopping on five days each week.	
Break your general goal into smaller, short-term goals.	In week 1, I will walk for at least 15 minutes a day without stopping for at least three of the next seven days.	
By what date do you want to accomplish this goal?	I want to accomplish my short-term goal by March 15 (seven days from now).	
How will you know when you have reached your goal? Identify the criteria you will use to determine that you have achieved your goal to your satisfaction.	I will use my watch to check the time. I will write the number of minutes that I walk each day on my calendar. I will also record my pulse and RPE. My RPE will be 12 to 13.	
What are you willing to do (or give up) to attain your goal? Be honest with yourself. Timing, motivation, and other factors will affect your ability to attain your goal.	I will get up 30 minutes earlier each morning so that I can walk before eating breakfast and getting dressed for the day. I will ask my spouse to walk with me.	
What is stopping you from achieving your goal? Try to identify the barriers and then develop strategies to overcome them. Commit to increasing your awareness of your motivators, limitations, expectations, and barriers. Reassess your goals regularly.	I will walk outside in the neighborhood if the weather is good. If the weather is poor when I get up, I will plan to drive to a nearby mall to walk after work.	

Write a Personal Contract

A personal contract is an effective tool for developing your exercise plan. The contract specifies everything that you will do. Use the information that you've gained in this chapter to write a contract with yourself to achieve your aerobic exercise goal. Complete the form in action box 9.3. Sign the contract to show your commitment to the plan. Involve another person in your plan by asking for his or her support and signature. Be specific about the type of support you want. Each week reevaluate your progress and rewrite your contract for the next week. Make an extra copy of the contract to use again in the future. A copy of a similar contract is in the appendix.

If you're not ready to make a plan for aerobic exercise, remember that you can use the personal contract to set a goal that keeps you moving forward. You might commit to talking with a friend who is active to find out how he or she started, or you might decide which sedentary activities you plan to replace with more active ones. You can record those types of things on the personal contract provided in the appendix.

Action Box 9.3: My Personal Contract

Example: Linda

For the week of February 12 (week 1), I, Linda, will do the following aerobic exercise.

Day	Type of activities and where I will exercise	Minutes
Sun., 12		
Mon., 13	Brisk walking in neighborhood	15
Tue., 14		
Wed., 15	Brisk walking in neighborhood	15
Thu., 16		
Fri., 17	Brisk walking in neighborhood	15
Sat., 18		

When I complete the listed activities, I will reward myself as follows: I will plan 45 minutes for a relaxing bubble bath.

I will involve John (my husband) in my plan as follows: I will ask John to walk with me.

Signed: Linda   Date: February 10

Witness: John   Date: February 10

Action Box 9.3:   My Personal Contract

For the week of _____ , I, (your name) _____

_____ , will engage in the following physical activities.

Day	Type of activities and where I will exercise	Minutes
Sunday		
Monday		
Tuesday		
Wednesday		
Thursday		
Friday		
Saturday		

When I complete the listed activities, I will reward myself as follows: _____

_____

I will involve _____ in my plan as follows: _____

_____

Signed:_____ Date:_____

Witness:_____ Date:_____

Check Your Progress

If you follow the model aerobic exercise plan that we have suggested, you will see results after only a few weeks. Here's a simple walking test you can do to check for improvement in your aerobic fitness. Do the test and fill in action box 9.4 with your baseline results. Repeat the test once every week or two and record your results. Nothing motivates like success.

■ Walk any course that takes you four to six minutes to complete. The course doesn't have to be flat, and you don't need to know the distance. You don't have to walk quickly or at any particular speed.

■ Record how long it takes you to walk the course to the nearest second. This number is your baseline.

■ Repeat the walking test after a few weeks of increased activity. Be sure to walk the same course that you walked in the baseline test. You should see changes. If you have improved your aerobic fitness, you should be able to walk the same course in a shorter time, or you should feel less tired if you walk at the same speed.

Action Box 9.4:   Are You Getting Fitter?

Record your times for the walking test. Be sure that you walk the same course each time you do the test.

Date of test	Time (minutes and seconds)	RPE or pulse rate	Notes
	Baseline		

Summary

In this chapter, you learned about the FITT (frequency, intensity, time, and type) plan and how to apply it to structured aerobic exercise. You also learned several ways to assess the intensity of your exercise (how hard you are working). We presented a model aerobic exercise program that you can use to develop your own program for periods of 6 weeks to 24 weeks. Use the models to set short- and long-term goals and commit to your goals with a personal contract. Start right away to implement your plan. Even before you start to see measurable results (and you will see results!), you will feel better about yourself. In the next chapter you will learn how to include the other fitness components in your structured exercise plan—strength building, flexibility exercises, and balance exercises—for a total fitness program.

Chapter Checklist

Following are some ways in which you can apply what you have learned in this chapter to your daily life. Over the next few days and weeks try to do as many of these activities as possible.

❑ If you are not taking a medicine that alters your heart rate, determine your training zone. Take your pulse while exercising to see whether you are within your training zone.

❑ Practice using the Borg scale of perceived exertion to rate the intensity of your exercise. Everyone can use this method of rating intensity.

❑ Develop your own aerobic fitness goal and program for an exercise of your choice. Use our model program as your guide.

❑ Write a personal contract to achieve a short-term aerobic fitness goal. Your contract should be for at least a week. You adjust your program each week. Remember to reward yourself! Stay with your program for at least 12 weeks before trying a different aerobic exercise.

❑ Do the simple walking test to get a baseline assessment of your fitness level.

❑ Continue to say affirmations about being physically active. Using affirmations is one of the best ways to keep yourself motivated.

Word Search

See if you can find 10 important words from this chapter in the grid that follows. Words appear forward and backward in rows, columns, and diagonals. The solution is shown on page 232.

```
Y R G F L T X Q C A V H I T F
Z J V W A R M U P M Q G C R U
C J H F M A N G H K T A E T Z
G I Q L S I W P I Y R Q A G U
Y Y K O A N T B P T U Y E F X
R I H Q Z I N E N E P J Q L C
N J R M W N S O N T A U M T T
W O E M J G C C I X W K L C I
O R V X M Z Y Y C T B K M S M
D Q Z A N O F P Q P R L V C E
L T L T G N D D J Q O E J E P
O N B R P E J M D O S S X U I
O L V W W O R C E Y B V S E K
C N H J U O P F C K C W U P V
Y T I S N E T N I W N I E M Z
```

Contract	Intensity	Training zone
Cool-down	Pulse	Type
Exertion	Time	Warm-up
Frequency		

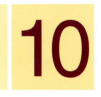

Add Strength, Balance, and Flexibility

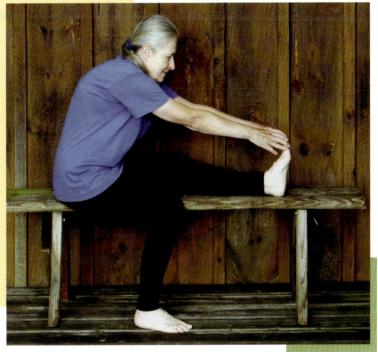

© Karlene V. Schwartz/Schwartz Search Gallery

In This Chapter

- ❑ Apply the FITT plan to strength-building and flexibility exercises.
- ❑ Learn how to do a variety of strength-building and balance exercises using body weight, handheld weights, resistance rubber bands, and weight machines.
- ❑ Include flexibility exercises, the most neglected type of exercise.
- ❑ Consider a sport or recreational activity.
- ❑ Use our model program for balanced fitness to plan your program.

Many people ask, "What is the best type of exercise?" No single kind of exercise is the best way to be physically active. Just as you need variety and balance in the foods you eat, you need a balanced fitness program to get the most benefit for your health. A balanced fitness program improves all areas of fitness: aerobic fitness, muscle fitness (strength and flexibility), and balance. To improve in all areas, you need to vary your activities throughout the week.

You might not be ready to do every type of physical activity. If that description fits you, use this chapter to learn more about how you can spice up your physical activity plans. You might find that you would enjoy adding an activity that improves your balance or flexibility to your lifestyle physical program. Maybe you'll choose to take the stairs, record your thoughts about physical activity, and do one balance activity this week. Set a goal that matches your stage of readiness to change.

Personal Profiles

Donna, Age 61

Donna has been an elementary school teacher for nearly 40 years. She hasn't missed work because of illness in several years. When she was younger she was an avid runner. Now she mostly walks for exercise, although at a brisk pace. She routinely logs 20 to 25 miles a week.

Jim, Age 59

Jim has worked in construction all his life. The activity of his job has helped keep him fit and trim. Besides getting physical activity on the job, Jim likes to work out with weights at home. He has set up a workout area in his garage. Almost every evening when he gets in from work, he changes clothes and heads to the garage for a few sets of heavy weightlifting before dinner. He's pretty proud of the way he looks.

Martin, Age 58

Martin, a computer software sales representative, had bypass surgery when he was 52. The episode changed his life. He gave up his inactive lifestyle. Now he rides a stationary cycle two or three days a week for 30 minutes at a time. He also works out with light dumbbells twice a week. To relieve stress, he works in his garden for several hours on weekends and looks for other ways to be active through lifestyle pursuits and recreation. You'll see him take the stairs instead of the elevator every chance he gets. Once a week he shoots baskets in the driveway with a neighbor.

Some people focus on only one type of fitness and neglect the others. For example, some people, like Donna, can achieve a high level of aerobic fitness but have poor muscle strength in their upper bodies. Others, like Jim, believe that because they are strong, they are healthy. Of the three people described, Martin has the most balanced fitness program. His physical activity program develops aerobic fitness, muscle strength and endurance, balance, and flexibility.

As you get older, balanced fitness is essential to good health, function, and quality of life. One of the best things about a balanced fitness program is that it provides variety. You don't become bored as you might if you did only one type of activity.

FITT Plan for Muscle Fitness and Flexibility

In chapter 9 you learned about aerobic fitness and the FITT plan. This chapter will show you how to add the other fitness areas—muscle strength and endurance, joint flexibility, and balance.

Before we discuss the FITT plan for muscle fitness, you need to know a few terms related to strength building and stretching exercises. These areas of fitness have a language all their own. See the following glossary and become familiar with any terms that are new to you.

Strength-Building and Stretching Glossary

body weight activities—Strength-building exercises that use the weight of the body and gravity as resistance.

flexibility—Ability to move a joint through its full range of motion; stretching improves flexibility.

muscle endurance—Ability of the muscle to make repeated contractions with a less than maximal load; doing a large number of repetitions with low resistance improves muscle endurance.

muscle strength—Ability of the muscle to apply force; strength-building exercises using heavy resistance build muscle strength.

progression—Gradual increase in the load or resistance applied to the muscle so that it becomes stronger.

range of motion—Angles and directions through which joints normally move.

repetitions (reps)—Number of times a particular exercise is repeated without pausing during a set.

resistance—Load, force, or weight applied against the muscle.

set—Group of repetitions performed without pausing; a brief period of rest is allowed between sets for muscles to recover.

Now that you know some of the terms, we can discuss the FITT plan for muscle fitness, summarized in table 10.1. You already know the basics: *F* means frequency, *I* means intensity, and *T* means time. The second *T* means type, and the types of strength-building exercises are described in the next section.

Regarding frequency, strength-building exercises are recommended at least two days per week. You can do stretching exercises as much as desired, but at least several days per week. For intensity, you can use the Borg scale for perceived exertion to rate your strength-building exercises. Review the RPE table in chapter 9 if necessary. If you are trying to build muscle strength, your intensity rating may be as high as 15 or 16 at the end of your session. If muscle endurance is your goal, then lower RPEs around 12 or 13 are fine. Of course, stretching is not intended to be an intense exercise. Stretches should be easy and comfortable to do. For strength-building exercises, *time* means the number of times that you repeat the exercise (reps) rather than the time in minutes. People over age 50 should use less weight or resistance and do more reps (10 to 15). For stretching exercises, *time* means the number of seconds that you hold the stretch and the number of times that you repeat the stretch.

Types of Strength-Building Exercises

You can do a variety of types of strength-building exercises as part of a structured exercise program. In this chapter, we will show you several

Table 10.1   FITT Plan for Muscle Fitness

	Muscle strength and endurance	Joint flexibility (stretching)
F—Frequency	At least two days per week. Don't do strength-building exercises with the same muscle group two days in a row. Allow one day of rest for muscles to recover.	Daily, especially as you cool down after aerobic exercise.
I—Intensity	Begin at a rating of perceived exertion (RPE) of 12 to 14 on the Borg scale. At the end of your last set of strength-training exercises, you may be at an RPE of 15 or 16 or even higher.	Stretch slowly and with full control, never to the point of pain. Don't bounce.
T—Time	Select at least one exercise to strengthen each of the major muscle groups: shoulders, back, arms, chest, abdominals, thighs, hamstrings, calves. Do at least one set of 10 to 15 repetitions of each exercise.	Gradually apply tension on the muscle, hold it for 10 to 20 seconds, and then slowly release. Repeat the stretch three to five times. As you gain experience, try to hold stretches for 30 seconds or longer.

exercises for each of the major muscle groups. You can choose the type of exercise that suits you best.

All strength-building exercises apply resistance or force to the muscle. Resistance can come from your body weight and gravity, handheld weights, resistance rubber bands, or weight machines. Your body doesn't know, or care, what type of resistance you use. For example, a push-up is a common body weight exercise for the chest and shoulders. You can also apply resistance to the chest and shoulders by exercising on a weight machine or by using handheld weights or resistance rubber bands. See the illustrations in figure 10.1. The positions and techniques are different, but each type of exercise will make chest and shoulder muscles stronger.

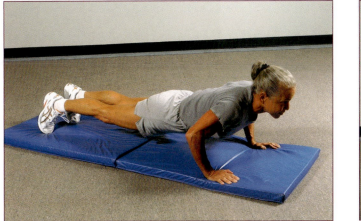

a

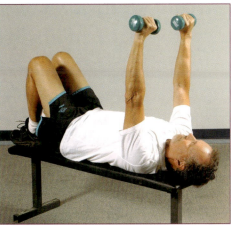

b

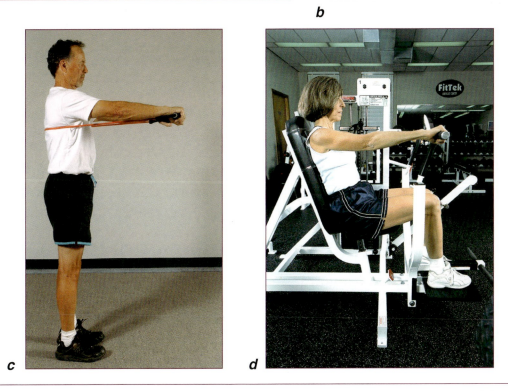

c   d

■ **Figure 10.1**   Exercises to strengthen the chest and shoulders: *(a)* push-ups, *(b)* chest press using dumbbells; *(c)* chest press with resistance bands; *(d)* chest press with weight machine.

You can also build strength by doing various lifestyle activities. Activities that involve pushing (a lawn mover, vacuum cleaner, furniture, or broom), dragging and pulling (a garden hose, wagon), lifting and carrying (a child, groceries, bucket), and digging and shoveling (dirt, snow) all build strength. Some people—such as carpenters, painters, mechanics, firemen, landscapers, and movers—have jobs that involve heavy physical work and help them build and maintain strong muscles.

Body Weight Activities

Body weight activities use no equipment. The weight of the body and gravity provide the resistance. You probably remember calisthenics from your physical education class in school; now we call these body weight activities. Jumping jacks, push-ups, sit-ups, and pull-ups are examples of body weight activities. Doing body weight activities has many advantages. They are easy to do. No costs are involved because no equipment is required. You can do body weight activities anywhere, anytime. For some muscle groups, such as abdominal muscles, body weight activities are the preferred type of exercise.

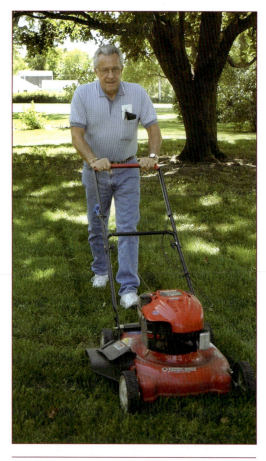

Pushing a lawn mower (not the self-propelled type) is an example of a lifestyle physical activity that strengthens the shoulders and chest.

Body weight activities also have some limitations. They rarely use all the major muscle groups. Some people think that body weight activities can be boring, so you may not stay motivated. The range of resistance is fixed by your weight. If you're heavy, body weight activities may be difficult. If you are inactive or have physical limitations, you may not have enough strength or may be physically unable to perform the exercise. If you have problems or injuries, body weight activities may cause more damage.

Handheld Weights and Resistance Rubber Bands

Handheld weights are sometimes called dumbbells. Handheld weights can range from 1 pound to 100 pounds (0.5 to 45 kilograms) or more. For our purposes we suggest that you use light handheld weights (less than 15 pounds or about 7 kilograms). You might need to start with a very light weight (2 pounds or 1 kilogram) and increase the weight as you grow stronger.

As their name suggests, resistance rubber bands are similar to large rubber bands. Resistance rubber bands are available in several forms. Some bands are long and flat with no handles. Others resemble ropes or cords. They may or may not have handles. Some bands are circles or loops. The thickness of the band determines the level of resistance—the thicker the band, the more resistance. Bands are also color coded by level of resistance. Select three different resistance levels that feel about right to you.

Handheld weights and resistance rubber bands are relatively inexpensive, so they are ideal for home use. You can store them easily and use them in a small space. Resistance rubber bands take up almost no space so they are easy to travel with. Another important advantage is that you can easily adjust handheld weights and resistance rubber bands to fit your strength level. But handheld weights and resistance bands have a few disadvantages. If you don't use the correct technique, you may not benefit fully from the exercise. A disadvantage of exercising with handheld weights and resistance bands is that the risk of injury is greater than it is when exercising on weight machines. You may need a helper, called a spotter, when using handheld weights. The role of the spotter is to ensure that you are using correct form, assist with lifts if you become tired, and motivate you to do your best.

Weight Machines

Popular at fitness centers, weight machines use pulleys or other mechanical systems to control the amount of weight that you lift. You typically sit on a seat or stand near a machine, adjust the amount of resistance, and then do the exercise. The weight is not freestanding.

Many kinds of weight machines have been designed for developing muscle fitness. If weight machines are available, you may enjoy using them. Machines are generally safer than handheld weights and body weight activities. You don't need a spotter. The major disadvantage is that you usually need to belong to a fitness center to use weight machines. Although weight machines are available for the home, they are expensive and take up a great deal of space.

Because most people go to a fitness center to use weight machines, we will not describe strength-building exercises using weight machines in this book. You can learn more about using weight machines in *Strength Training Past 50* (Westcott and Baechle 1998; available at www.HumanKinetics.com). Most fitness centers have fitness professionals available to show you how to use the machines if you are just getting started. Besides teaching you how to adjust and use the machines, your trainer will recommend specific machines for you to use, the sequence in which you should do the exercises, and the amount of resistance to use. Most fitness centers provide logs for recording your strength-building sessions. After you learn to adjust the seat and weights, the technique is easy to master. See the general strength-building techniques and tips on page 163. Here are a few specific tips for using machine machines:

- Wipe the cushions on the machine before and after use.
- Do not jerk the weights or let them drop.
- Remember the positions of the seats for future exercise session.

Exercises to Improve Balance

Although balance exercises are not technically a type of strength-building exercise, the overlap between the two is substantial. You can often modify a strength-building exercise to improve your balance. For example, all the strength-building exercises for the legs described in this chapter are also balance exercises. These exercises tell you to hold on to a table or chair for balance. Begin by holding with both hands or only one hand. As you progress, try holding with only one fingertip. Next, try these exercises without holding on at all. See how the hip flexion exercise on page 167 is modified to improve balance. Use these same techniques to modify other leg exercises to serve as balance exercises. You can also do the "anytime, anywhere" balance exercises as often as you like. See action box 10.1 for an easy way to check for improvements in your balance.

"Anytime, Anywhere" Balance Exercises

All you need to do these exercises is something sturdy to hold on to if you become unsteady. These exercises are adapted from *Exercise: A Guide From the National Institute on Aging* (National Institutes of Health n.d.). You can do these exercises as often as you like.

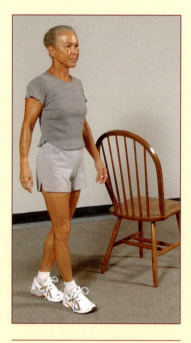

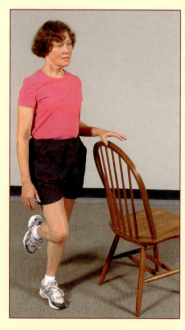

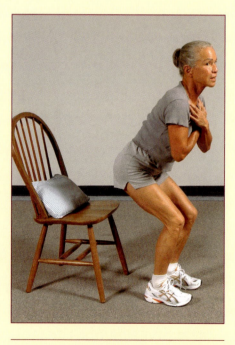

Walk heel to toe. Position your heel just in front of the toes of the opposite foot each time you take a step. Your heel and toes should touch or almost touch.

Stand on one foot. Alternate feet. You can do this exercise while you are waiting in line.

Sit forward in a straight-back chair. Stand up and sit down without using your hands.

Action Box 10.1: Is Your Balance Improving?

Here is an easy way to see whether your balance is improving. Time yourself as you stand on one foot without support for as long as possible. Be sure to stand near something sturdy to hold on to in case you lose your balance. Record the time. Repeat the test while standing on the other foot. Record your time. Test yourself again after one month. If your balance is improving, the time that you can stand on each foot should increase.

	Baseline	Month 1	Month 2	Month 3	Month 4	Month 5
Time standing on right foot						
Time standing on left foot						

General Strength-Building Techniques and Tips

The techniques and tips provided here apply to any type of strength-building exercise that you might do. Form and technique are important. You may do many repetitions, but if your technique is poor, your effort may be for naught and you may even be injured. Always follow these guidelines to get the best results from the strength-building exercises that you do.

■ If you have had hip replacement, other surgeries, or injuries, talk with your doctor or a physical therapist about appropriate strength-building exercises.

■ Wear comfortable shoes with rubber soles to provide secure footing.

■ Wear light, loose-fitting clothing to give you freedom of movement and allow the body to cool. Don't wear ties, scarves, jewelry, or anything that can be caught in resistance rubber bands, weights, or machines.

■ Use a minimum amount of resistance in the first few weeks. Gradually build up the weight. Starting out with weights that are too heavy can cause injuries.

■ Breathe in and out normally—out as you lift or push and in as you relax. Don't hold your breath. Holding your breath can cause your blood pressure to increase, decrease blood flow to the brain, and cause dizziness and fainting.

■ Take your time. Do each repetition of an exercise through the full range of motion. Use slow, controlled movements.

■ Exercise the larger muscles first (quadriceps, back, chest) and then the smaller muscles (hamstrings, calves, shoulders, biceps, triceps, and abdominals). The small muscles are always involved in the movements of the larger muscles. If you exercise the small muscles first and they become too tired, you won't be able to do the exercises that build the larger muscles. The quadriceps (front of the thighs) are the largest muscles in the legs. The back and chest muscles are the largest muscles in the upper part of the body.

■ Do at least one complete set of all exercises before repeating the exercises. This method allows you to work every muscle group at least once and provides a period of rest for each muscle before you exercise it again.

■ A set is 10 to 15 repetitions completed without pausing. Begin the exercise slowly with low resistance or weight. You should be able to do 10 repetitions of one set using good form. If you can't do at least 8 repetitions in a row, the weight is too heavy for you. When you are able to do 15 or more repetitions in a row, the weight is too light for you. Increase the resistance or weight by a small amount (two to five pounds, or one to two kilograms) or to a level of resistance at which you can do 10 repetitions without pausing. Work back up to 15 repetitions. When you can do a complete set at the new weight, increase the weight again. This process of gradually adding weight as your strength increases is called progression. You won't benefit from the strength exercise unless you overload your muscles.

■ When you can do two complete sets of 10 to 15 reps at an RPE of 14 to 15 ("hard"), stay at that level for maintenance of muscle strength and endurance. You can change the order of the exercises for variety.

■ Rest for 30 to 60 seconds after each set. This rest period is a good time to perform a few stretches with the muscle that you just worked.

■ Avoid locking the joints in your arms and legs in a tightly straightened position.

■ Never exercise the same muscle group on consecutive days. Muscles need a day of rest between exercise sessions. You can do strength-building exercises every day if you exercise muscles in the upper body on one day and muscles in the lower body on the next.

■ None of the exercises that you do should cause pain. Muscle soreness lasting up to a few days and slight fatigue are normal after doing strength-building exercises. If you feel exhausted, have sore joints, or pulled muscles, you are overdoing it.

■ Keep a record of your strength-building sessions. For each exercise, record the level of resistance, number of repetitions, number of sets, and other appropriate notes.

Using Body Weight, Handheld Weights, and Resistance Rubber Bands

This section includes several examples of strength-building exercises for the major muscle groups. Many of the exercises are based on those found in *Exercise: A Guide From the National Institute on Aging* (National Institutes of Health n.d.). You can begin with no added weight at all (only your body weight) and then add handheld weights as you get stronger. Exercises using resistance rubber bands are also shown for some of the muscle groups. Keep these tips in mind when using handheld weights or resistance rubber bands.

- Don't jerk or let your body sway.
- Count, "One, two" as you raise the weights and "One, two" as you lower them.
- When lifting weights from the floor, use your legs rather than your lower back to avoid injury to your back.
- If using handheld weights at a fitness center, be sure to return the weights to the rack when you have finished your exercise.
- If you wrap a resistance rubber band around any part of your body, be sure that it is not too tight.
- Always begin with thinner bands and gradually work up to thicker bands that provide more resistance.
- Don't let a band snap back. Always keep some tension on the band as you return to the starting position.

Exercises for Legs and Hips

These exercises improve strength, flexibility, and balance and assist in daily activities such as climbing stairs, walking, bending to lift or pick up objects, going to the toilet, housekeeping, gardening, and getting in and out of a chair, tub, or car. They also help prevent low back pain. See action box 10.2 for an easy test to measure improvements in your lower-body strength.

Action Box 10.2: Are Your Legs Getting Stronger?

Here's an easy way to know whether your legs are getting stronger. Time yourself as you walk up a flight of stairs (at least 10 steps) as fast as you can safely. Record the time as your baseline. Repeat the test, using the same stairs, one month later. If you have improved your lower-body strength, you should be able to walk up the stairs in a shorter time.

(continued)

	Baseline	Month 1	Month 2	Month 3	Month 4	Month 5
Time to walk up a flight of stairs						

Chair Stand (Thighs and Abdomen)

The first part of this exercise works your abdominal muscles.

1. Place a small pillow against the back of a chair.

2. Sit in the middle or toward the front of the chair, with knees bent and feet flat on the floor.

3. Lean back on the pillow in a half-reclining position with your hands crossed over your chest.

4. Use your abdominal muscles to raise your upper body forward until you are sitting upright, using your hands as little as possible.

The second part of this exercise works your thigh muscles.

5. Slowly stand up, using your hands as little as possible. Slowly sit back down.

6. Keep your back and shoulders straight throughout the exercise.

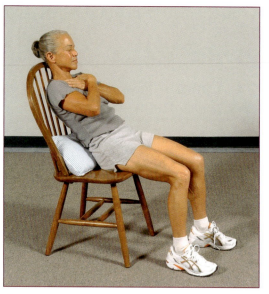

a

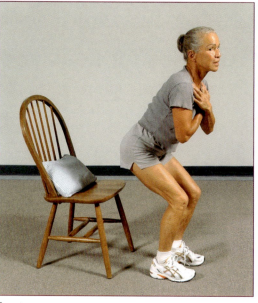

b

Chair stand: *(a)* strengthens abdominal muscles; *(b)* strengthens thigh muscles.

Hip Flexion
(Hips and Front of Thighs)

1. Stand straight, holding a tall, stable object for balance (such as the back of a chair).

2. Slowly bend one knee toward the chest without bending the waist or hips.

3. Hold the position for two counts.

4. Slowly lower the leg to the floor.

5. Repeat with the other leg.

As you progress, add the modifications shown below to your leg exercises to improve your balance.

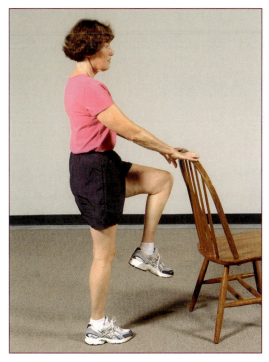

Hip flexion as described.

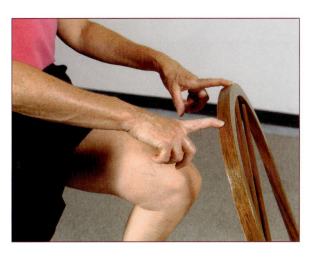

a

Hip flexion with modifications to improve balance: *(a)* Holding chair with one fingertip; *(b)* without holding (no hands).

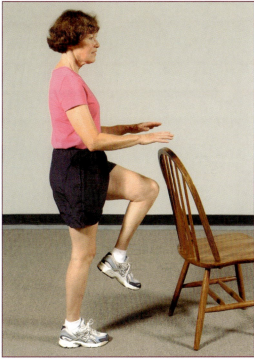

b

Hip Extension (Buttocks and Lower Back)

1. Stand about 12 to 18 inches (30 to 45 centimeters) from a table or chair.

2. Bend forward at hips while holding on to table or chair.

3. Slowly lift one leg straight backward. Be sure that the movement comes from the hip joint, not the back.

4. Hold the position.

5. Slowly lower your leg to the floor.

6. Repeat with the other leg.

Variation: You can also do hip extension exercises with looped resistance bands. Place the band around your ankles or, for less resistance around your thighs, just above your knees.

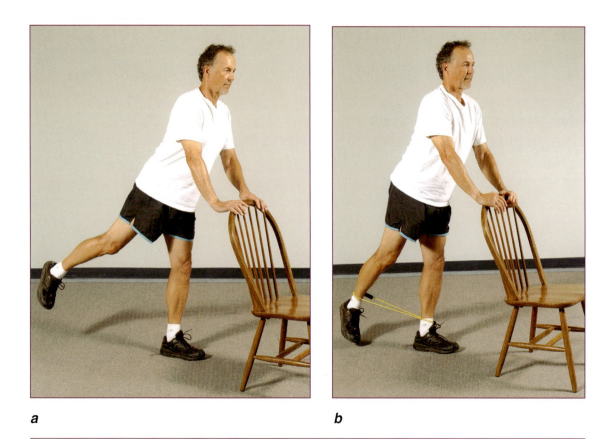

a   b

Hip extension (a) in standard position; (b) with looped resistance rubber band for added resistance.

Knee Extension (Front of Thighs and Shins)

1. Sit in a straight-back chair. Only your toes and the balls of your feet should be resting on the floor. If you need to raise your knees, form a roll with a bath towel and place it under your knees.

2. Rest your hands on your knees or the sides of the chair.

3. Slowly extend one leg to straighten your knee as much as possible. Point your toes forward.

4. Hold position and flex your foot to point your toes back toward your head.

5. Slowly lower your leg back to the floor.

6. Repeat with the other leg.

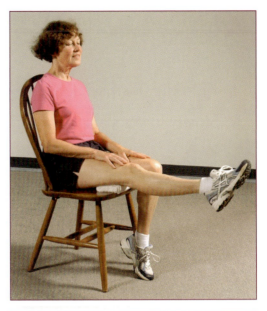

Knee extension.

Knee Flexion (Back of Thighs)

1. Standing tall, hold a table or back of a chair for balance.

2. Slowly bring your heel up toward your buttocks. Don't move your upper leg at all. Bend only your knee.

3. Hold the position.

4. Slowly lower your foot to the floor.

5. Repeat with the other leg.

6. Add modifications to improve balance.

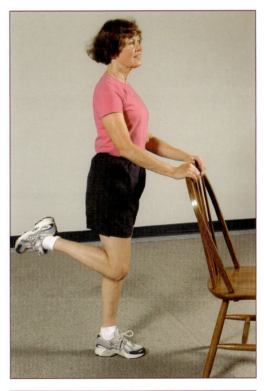

Knee flexion.

Side Leg Raise (Sides of Hips and Thighs)

1. Standing tall, hold a table or back of a chair for balance. Place your feet slightly apart. Contract your abdominal muscles.

2. Slowly lift one leg to the side about 6 to 12 inches (15 to 30 centimeters).

3. Hold the position.

4. Slowly lower your leg.

5. Keep your back and both knees straight, but not locked, throughout the exercise.

6. Repeat with the other leg.

7. Add a looped resistance rubber band when you are ready.

8. Add modifications to improve balance.

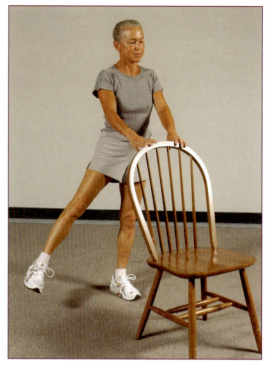

Side leg raise.

Calf Raise (Ankle and Calf Muscles)

1. Stand straight, holding a table or chair for balance.

2. Slowly stand on your tiptoes, as high as possible.

3. Hold the position.

4. Slowly lower your heels to the floor.

5. Do the exercise standing on one leg only, alternating legs as your strength improves.

Exercises for Back, Shoulders, Chest, and Arms

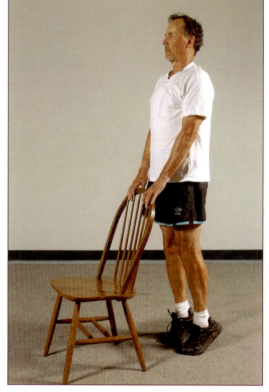

Calf raise.

This series of exercises improves strength, flexibility, mobility, and function of the upper body. Doing these exercises will help you perform many daily activities including lifting or reaching objects above your head, carrying groceries, vacuuming and sweeping, holding children and pets, bathing, using the toilet, dressing, grooming, preparing and eating meals, and driving.

Shoulder Flexion (Shoulders)

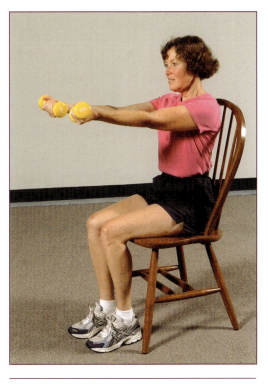

1. Sit in a chair with your feet flat on floor. Keep your feet even with your shoulders.

2. Begin with your arms straight down at your sides with your palms turned inward.

3. Raise both arms in front of you to shoulder height. Keep both arms straight and rotate so that your palms face upward.

4. Hold the position.

5. Slowly lower your arms to your sides.

6. Add handheld weights when you are ready.

Shoulder flexion with handheld weights.

Arm Raise (Shoulders)

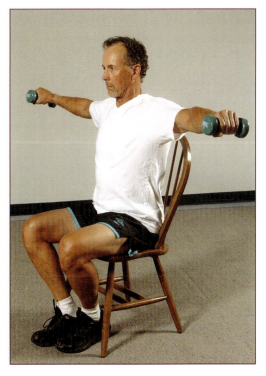

1. Sit in a chair with your feet flat on the floor. Keep your feet even with your shoulders.

2. Begin with your shoulders relaxed, your arms straight down at your sides, and your palms turned inward.

3. Raise both arms to the sides to shoulder height. Keep both arms straight with palms down.

4. Hold the position.

5. Slowly lower your arms to your sides.

6. Add handheld weights (not too heavy) when you are ready.

Arm raise with handheld weights.

Side Shoulder Raise (Shoulders) With Resistance Rubber Band

1. While standing or sitting, place your foot on one end of the band and grip the other end of the band with your opposite hand.

2. Start with your arm by your side with the palm of your hand facing inward.

3. With your elbow slightly bent, raise your arm to your side to shoulder level

4. Slowly lower your arm to the starting position.

5. Repeat with the other arm.

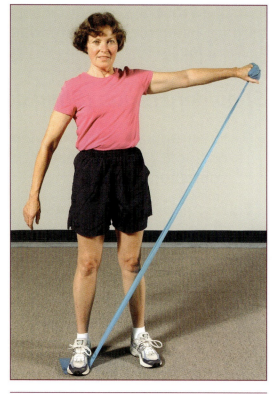

Side shoulder raise with resistance rubber band.

Variation: A variation of this exercise is the front shoulder raise. For this version, the band goes under the foot on the same side of your body as the arm that you will raise. Raise your arm in front of your body.

Chest Fly (Chest Muscles)

1. Lie flat on the floor (prone position).

2. Hold weights in each hand.

3. Bring your hands together at chest height with your palms facing inward. Your elbows should be slightly bent in a semicircular position.

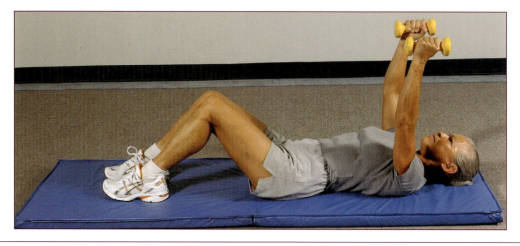

a

Chest fly with handheld weights: *(a)* upper or closed position *(continued);*

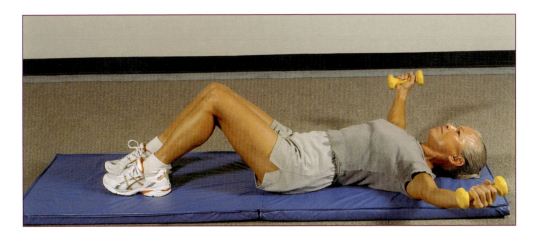

b

... *(b)* lower or open position.

4. Open your arms until your elbows are even with your shoulders.

5. Hold the position.

6. Close your arms (like hugging a tree) so that your hands are together again.

Chest Press (Chest) With Resistance Rubber Band

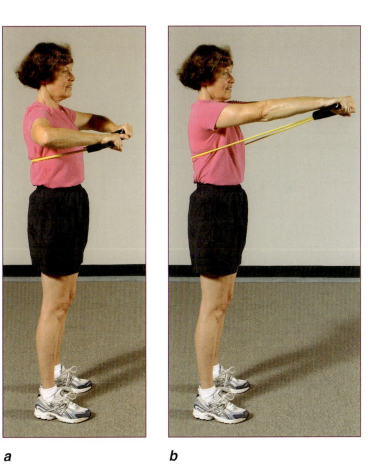

1. Grip the ends of the band in each hand. Place the band behind your upper back.

2. Bend your elbows to a 90-degree angle and lift your arms so that they are parallel to the floor. Press your arms forward until they are straight.

3. Slowly bend your elbows and return to the starting position.

4. Keep your wrists straight at all times.

a   *b*

Chest press with resistance rubber band: *(a)* band behind upper back; *(b)* arms pressed forward.

Seated Row (Upper Back, Shoulders, and Neck) With Resistance Rubber Band

1. Sit up straight on the floor with your legs straight in front of you.

2. Grip one end of the band in each hand. Loop the band all the way around your feet for safety.

3. Extend your arms in front of you with your shoulders relaxed and your palms facing each other.

4. Contract your abdominal muscles while pulling both ends of the band toward your hips. Pull the elbows back so that you squeeze the shoulder blades together.

5. Slowly return your hands to the starting position and repeat.

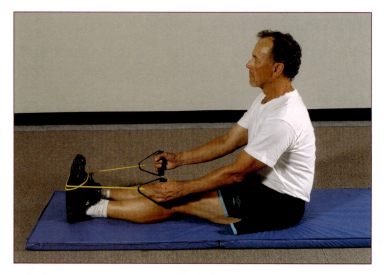

a

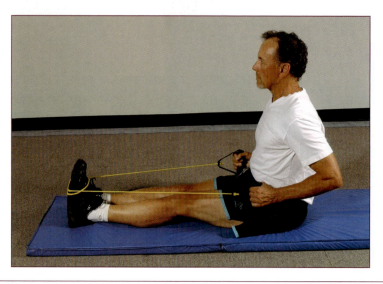

b

Seated row with resistance rubber bands: *(a)* band looped around feet; *(b)* pulling ends of band toward the hips.

Biceps Curl (Front of Upper Arms) With Handheld Weights

1. Sit forward on the edge of an armless chair with your back straight.

2. Place your feet flat on the floor with your feet shoulder-width apart.

3. Hold hand weights at your side with your arms straight and your palms turned inward.

4. Slowly bend one elbow, lifting the weight toward your chest. Rotate your palm to face your shoulder while lifting the weight.

5. Contract your abdominal muscles while doing the exercise.

6. Hold the position.

7. Slowly lower your arm to starting position.

8. Repeat with the other arm.

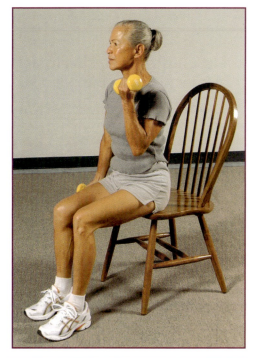

Biceps curl with handheld weights.

Triceps Extension (Back of Upper Arms) With Handheld Weights

1. Sit forward on the edge of a chair with your back straight.

2. Place your feet flat on the floor with your feet shoulder-width apart.

3. While holding a hand weight, raise one arm straight

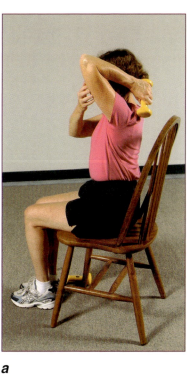

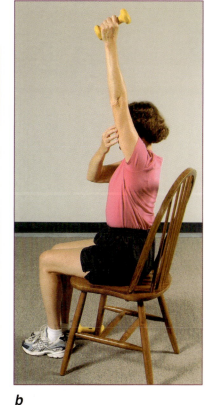

a   *b*

Triceps extension with handheld weights: *(a)* elbow bent with weight toward shoulder; *(b)* elbow straight with weight toward ceiling.

toward the ceiling. Use your other hand to support this arm below the elbow.

4. Bend the raised arm at the elbow, bringing the hand weight back toward the shoulder.

5. Slowly straighten the arm toward the ceiling.

6. Hold the position.

7. Repeat, slowly bending your arm toward your shoulder again.

Biceps Curl (Front of Upper Arms) With Resistance Rubber Band

1. Stand with both feet on the center of the band. Grip the ends of the band with your hands.

2. Start with your arms down by your side with the palms of your hands facing up. Keep your elbows close to your body.

3. Bend your arms so that your fists curl upward to your shoulders.

4. Slowly lower your arms.

This exercise can also be performed by alternating arms.

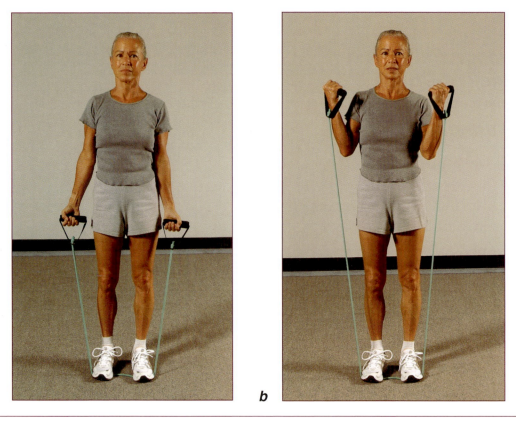

a   *b*

Biceps curl with resistance rubber band: *(a)* band under feet with arms down; *(b)* arms curled to shoulders.

Triceps Extension (Back of Upper Arms)
With Resistance Rubber Band

1. Place your foot on one end of the band. Grip the other end of the band with your hand on the opposite side of your body. Take one step back with your other foot.

2. Bend your front knee slightly. Rest your free hand on your hip.

3. Place the hand holding the band against your hip with the palm facing down.

4. Slowly straighten your arm out behind you.

5. Slowly return your hand to your hip.

6. Repeat with the other arm.

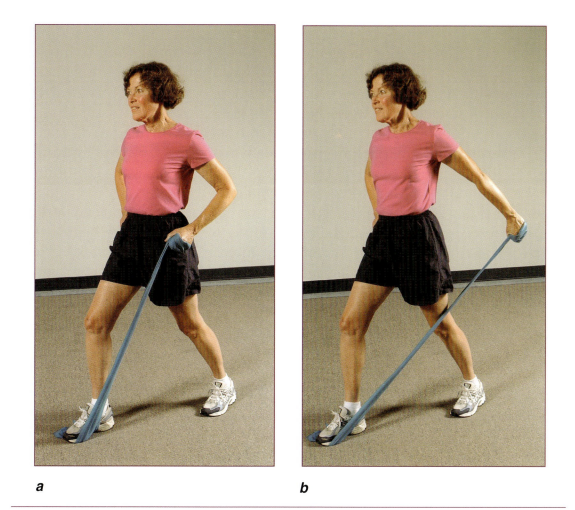

a   *b*

Triceps curl with resistance rubber band: *(a)* band under foot with bended knee and hand at hip; *(b)* arm straightened behind the back

If You Have Arthritis

Before you start to exercise, massage the stiff or sore areas or apply heat treatments to the area that you will be exercising. Heat relaxes your joints and muscles and helps relieve pain. Cold also reduces pain and swelling for some people. Cold is usually applied after the exercise session. You can apply heat or cold in many ways, including the following:

- Take a warm (not hot) shower before you exercise.

- Apply a heating pad or hot pack to the sore area.

- Sit in a warm whirlpool for a few minutes.

- Wrap a bag of ice or frozen vegetables in a towel and place it on the sore area.

Stretching

Flexibility is often the most neglected part of a fitness program. To improve flexibility, you need to do stretching exercises regularly. Stretching can be the easiest and most enjoyable type of exercise to perform. You can stretch almost every muscle of your body. Having good flexibility means that you have the freedom of movement to do the things that you need to do and like to do. Stretching exercises alone, however, will not improve your endurance or strength. You need to do all three—aerobic exercise, strength-building exercises, and flexibility exercises—for balanced fitness.

Besides doing stretches as part of your exercise program, you can perform gentle stretches at other times. For example, when you have been sitting for a long period, stretching the muscles in your shoulders, back, or neck feels good. Stretching and massaging tense muscles are important stress management techniques.

Stretching Techniques and Tips

For many years, trainers encouraged people to stretch cold muscles vigorously to loosen up before activity. In recent years, stretching exercises to warm up have fallen out of favor because they may cause injuries. If you are stretching before exercise, stretch only lightly and briefly. Wait to do intense stretching until after a few minutes of aerobic exercise. Stretching after physical activity helps the muscles relax and return to their resting state. Muscles are easier to stretch after physical activity because they are looser. Always follow these guidelines to get the best results from the stretches that you do.

- If you have had hip replacement, other surgeries, or injuries, talk with your doctor or a physical therapist about appropriate stretching exercises.

- If you are doing only stretching exercises on a particular day, do a little bit of easy walking while pumping your arms to warm up. Stretching your muscles too hard before they are warmed up may result in injury.

- As you move into the stretch, maintain tension on the muscle. Hold the stretch for 10 to 20 seconds and then slowly release. As you gain experience, try to hold the stretch for 30 to 60 seconds.

- Relax between stretches and then repeat. Try to reach a little farther with each stretch.

- Do each stretching exercise three to five times at each session. Your goal is to perform each stretch slowly and carefully, maintaining control from beginning to end.

- Never stretch to the point of pain. A mild pulling sensation is normal.

- Don't bounce while the muscle is fully stretched. Bouncing can cause injury.

- Breathe normally. Take full, slow breaths during a stretch. Fill your lungs completely. Feel your diaphragm move. When you inhale you can increase the stretch slightly. Exhale while you hold the stretch.

- Avoid locking your joints into place when you straighten them during stretches. Your arms and legs should be straight when you stretch them, but don't lock them in a tightly straight position. Keep your joints slightly bent while stretching.

Getting Up From the Floor

If you are concerned that you might have difficulty getting up from the floor, invite someone to exercise with you. You can assist each other, if needed. Here are some tips to help you get into a lying position and get back up.

To lie on the floor:

1. Stand next to a sturdy chair that won't tip over. Put the chair against a wall, if necessary.

2. Put your hands on the seat of the chair.

3. Lower yourself down on one knee.

4. Bring the other knee down.

5. Put your left hand on the floor and lean on it as you bring your left hip to the floor.

6. Your weight is now on your left hip. Straighten your legs out.

7. Lie on your left side and roll onto your back.

To get up from the floor:

1. Roll onto your left side.

2. Place your right hand on the floor at about the level of your ribs to push your shoulders off the floor.

3. Your weight is on your left hip.

4. Roll forward onto your knees, leaning on both hands for support.

5. Place your hands on the seat of the chair that you used to lie down.

6. Lift one of your knees so that one leg is bent with your foot flat on the floor.

7. Lean onto the chair for support and rise from this position.

Note: You can also do this movement from your right side.

Personal Profile

George, Age 56

At his most recent physical exam, George complained to his doctor about frequent joint stiffness and soreness. He was surprised to learn that he had arthritis. Although he knew that arthritis was common in older people, he thought he was too young to have developed the condition. Along with medication, pain management, and other parts of his treatment program, his doctor prescribed regular exercise. She emphasized the many health benefits of exercise but really got George's attention when she explained what could happen if he didn't exercise. Without exercise, the doctor said that his joints would likely become more stiff and painful. Muscles would become smaller and weaker, and bones would become more brittle. Joints that stayed bent in one position for too long (without movement) might not be able to be straightened out. George might even lose the use of those joints. Sometimes, George has been tempted to avoid exercise, especially when he was experiencing a flare-up of his arthritis symptoms. But he is committed to a regular, balanced fitness program. He participates in a water aerobics class or rides a stationary cycle and follows that with stretching. He also does strength-building exercises with light dumbbells and resistance rubber bands. So far, he has managed his arthritis well. One of the best benefits of regular exercise has been avoiding the depression that comes with the pain of arthritis.

Stretches for Major Muscle Groups and Joints

This section includes examples of stretches for the major muscle groups and joints. Many of the exercises are based on those found in *Exercise: A Guide From the National Institute on Aging* (National Institutes of Health n.d.).

Hamstring Stretch (Back of Thighs)

1. Sit sideways on a bench or other hard surface (such as two chairs placed side by side). Stretch one leg out straight on the bench. Your other leg is off the bench with your foot on the floor.

2. Lean forward from the hips (not your waist) until you feel stretching in the leg on the bench. Keep your back and shoulders straight.

3. Hold the stretch while contracting the abdominal muscles.

4. Relax and repeat with the other leg.

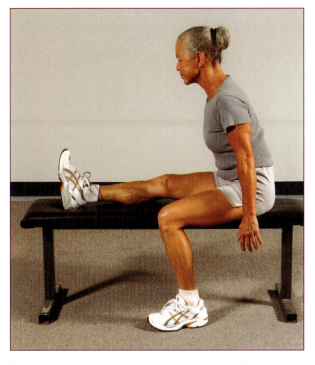

Hamstring stretch.

Calf Stretch (Lower Legs)

1. Stand with your hands on a wall with arms straight at shoulder level.

2. Step back 1 to 2 feet (30 to 60 centimeters), keeping one leg straight. The knee of the other leg is bent. Both feet are flat on the floor.

3. If you don't feel a stretch, move your back foot farther from the wall until you feel the stretch in your calf.

4. Keep one knee straight and hold the position.

5. Repeat with the other leg.

Note: You can also do this stretch with both knees bent. A light calf stretch is appropriate before you start to walk or jog.

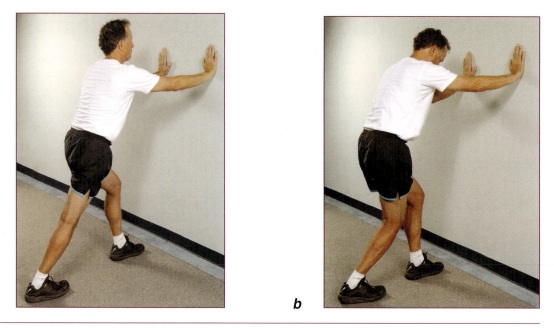

Calf stretch: *(a)* with back knee straight; *(b)* with both knees bent.

Triceps Stretch (Back of Upper Arms)

1. Hold a towel in your right hand.

2. Raise your right arm and bend your elbow to drape the towel down your back.

3. Grasp the bottom end of the towel with your left hand.

4. Climb your left hand higher up the towel an inch or two (two to five centimeters) at a time. (This action pulls your right arm down, causing the stretch.) Continue to climb your left hand as high as possible.

5. Reverse the positions and repeat the stretch.

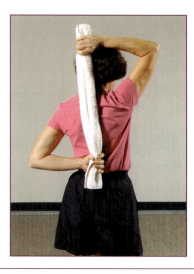
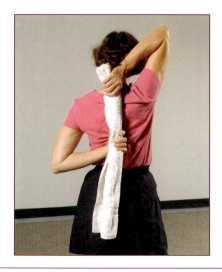

Triceps stretch: *(a)* beginning position; *(b)* left hand climbing up the towel.

Wrist Stretch

1. Place your hands together in front of you in a praying position, hands flat against each other.

2. Slowly raise your elbow until your arms are parallel to the floor. Keep your hands flat against each other.

3. Hold the position, then repeat.

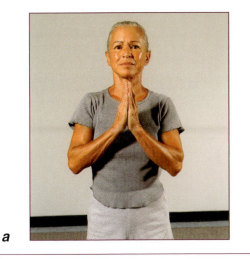 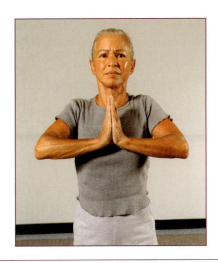

a   b

Wrist stretch: *(a)* hands in praying position; *(b)* hands with elbows raised.

Leg and Back Stretch

1. Lie on your back on the floor with your legs extended in front of you.

2. Bend one knee and raise it slowly toward your chest. Use both hands to hold your raised leg at the knee and pull toward you.

3. Hold the position.

4. Return the leg to the extended position and repeat the stretch with the other leg

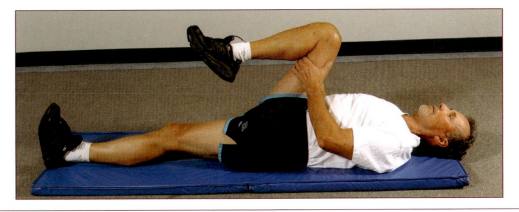

Leg and back stretch.

Arched Back Stretch

1. Kneel on your hands and knees with your back straight. Let your head hang down.

2. Keeping your head down, arch your back, feeling the pull from the shoulders to your lower back.

3. Hold the position and then return to your starting position.

4. Repeat the stretch.

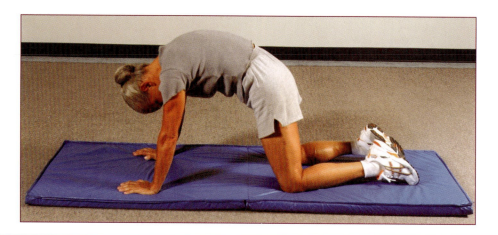

Arched back stretch.

Upper Back and Arm Stretch

1. Sit in a chair with your back straight.

2. Reach up with both arms, interlacing your fingers with your palms upward.

3. Reach as high as you can, keeping your back and neck straight.

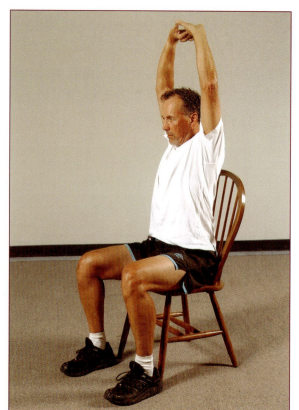

Upper back and arm stretch.

Neck Stretch

1. Stand with your hands on your hips and your feet about shoulder-width apart.

2. Slowly rotate your head to the left. Keep your chin level with the floor. Do not tilt your head. Hold the position.

3. Rotate your head to the right. Hold the position.

4. Caution: Do not tilt your head back while doing this exercise.

5. Repeat the stretches.

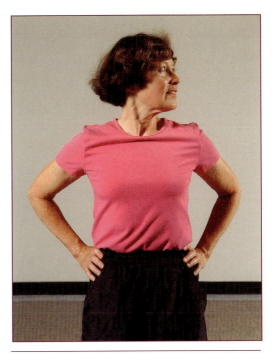

Neck stretch. You can also do this stretch while seated or lying.

Trunk Stretch

1. Stand with your feet about shoulder-width apart and your back straight.

2. Put your right hand on your right hip.

3. While contracting your abdominal muscles, raise your left hand over your head with the elbow slightly bent.

4. Bend your body to the right, arching your left arm over your head.

5. Repeat the stretch on your right side.

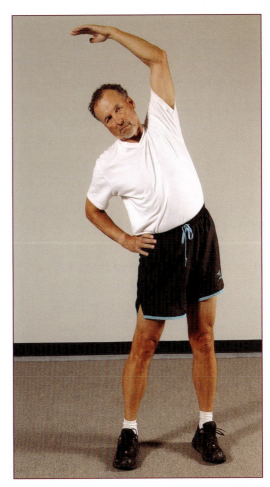

Trunk stretch.

Sports for Active Older Adults

Many people over age 50 participate in sports and recreational activities. As part of a balanced fitness program, sports and recreational activities have much to recommend them:

- Participating in sports is an excellent way to stay physically active. Many active sports count as exercise. Energy expended through sports improves your overall fitness and helps you control your weight. Because you're also having fun, sports don't seem like exercise. You are more likely to stay motivated and participate. Time flies, and you may barely notice the effort.

- As you begin to focus on the strategy and tactics of the game, you let go of stress. Participation in sports helps with stress management and increases self-esteem and personal satisfaction.

- You can plan opportunities for social activities with family and friends around sports. When you are traveling or on vacation, sports and recreational activities give you access to new friends and local culture that you would otherwise not encounter. You will meet others who share your values and interests.

You may be thinking, "I can't play sports. Sports are for athletes." Although some sports are best left to younger or more athletic people, you can be involved in many sports and recreational activities throughout your lifetime. Each year, thousands of people in their 70s, 80s, and 90s participate in the Senior Olympics. Events include sports from basketball to sprinting to race walking.

As people get older, many don't participate in sports because they think that the risk is too high. Remember, however, that risk is a relative term. You face some risk every day getting in and out of your car, walking across the parking lot, or venturing out to shop for groceries. These types of risk are known and accepted.

Each sport or recreational activity carries risk. The level of risk varies from very low (walking or golf) to very high (skating or downhill skiing). The risk of injury, in general, increases with the speed of movement, likelihood and consequences of falling, and amount of body contact. All risk is relative and depends on the sport and on your level of skill, physical conditioning, and experience.

Regardless of the sport you choose, think about what is required and use good judgment to manage risk and enjoy yourself without harm or injury. For example, if you participate in a brisk walking program on a track at the neighborhood school, your risk of injury is low. But if you go hiking in a remote mountainous area with difficult access, your risk is much higher. Even if you are an experienced hiker conditioned to high altitude, have the right kind of gear, and know the environment, you're at greater risk than you would be on the high school track. But because you are active and fit, your risk is lower than it would be for someone who is unfit and inexperienced.

Find the sport that interests you. Evaluate your motivation, skills, conditioning, and resources to decide which sport is right for you. Use the questions in action box 10.3 to evaluate some popular sports and recreational activities. After you have identified a sport of interest to you, make plans to find out how to become involved.

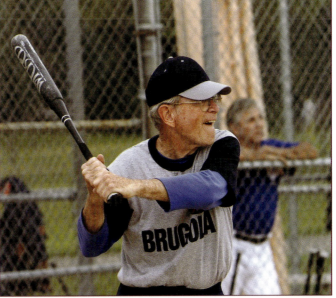

Sports such as softball are a healthy outlet for competition. The social aspects of team sports make them fun for participants and spectators alike.

Action Box 10.3: Pick a Sport or Recreational Activity

Answer the questions for these activities or other activities of interest to you. The more yes answers you give, the more likely it is that the activity is a good choice for you.

	Golf	Tennis	Softball	Hiking	Biking	Dancing	Other
Do you have the necessary knowledge and skills?							
Are you in good enough shape? • Aerobic fitness • Strength • Flexibility • Balance • Coordination							
Is your risk of injury relatively low?							

(continued)

	Golf	Tennis	Softball	Hiking	Biking	Dancing	Other
Is the place where you will participate in the sport convenient?							
Do you have the equipment?							
Can you afford the cost to participate?							
Would you enjoy the social aspects of the sport?							

Some people enjoy competition, and sports are a healthy way to compete. But you don't have to compete with others. You can compete with yourself by including sports-related goals as part of your overall fitness program.

Many people participate in road races, fun walks, or fun runs without trying to beat the clock. Their goal is only to enjoy the fellowship, finish the race, get the T-shirt, and feel good about their accomplishments. Others enter sponsored events to raise money for charity. Even if you are not interested in competition, you could end up a winner.

Personal Profile

Fran, Age 81

Fran entered a walking event to support breast cancer research. She was surprised when her name was called as a winner in the over-70 group. She won second place in a group of fewer than 10 participants in her age category and finished ahead of many participants who were decades younger.

Model Program for Balanced Fitness

In chapter 9 we provided a model program for aerobic fitness following the FITT plan. But, as you learned, aerobic fitness is not the only type of fitness important for people over age 50. Muscle strength and endurance, balance, and flexibility are as important as aerobic fitness, maybe even

Table 10.2   Suggested Types of Structured Exercise

Aerobic exercises	Strength-building exercises	Balance exercises	Flexibility exercises
Walking Water activities Stationary cycling	Body weight activities Handheld weights Resistance rubber bands Weight machines	"Anytime, anywhere" balance exercises Strength exercises with modifications	Stretches

more important, as you get older. These other types of fitness keep you functioning and independent. When you add exercise to improve muscle and joint fitness to your aerobic exercise program, you will have a total balanced fitness program.

Choose the specific exercises that you prefer from the various types that have been introduced (table 10.2). Our model programs for balanced fitness are described in table 10.3. The beginning balanced fitness program shows the frequency (F) of various types of exercise. The beginning program starts with three days of structured aerobic exercise and two days of strength-building exercise. Let's suppose that walking is your choice for aerobic exercise. By looking at the "Beginning" column of table 10.3, you can see that you would plan to walk three days (Monday, Wednesday, and Friday). You would follow the intensity (I) and time (T) guidelines recommended in chapter 9. On Tuesday and Thursday, you would do at least one strength-building exercise for each of the major muscle groups (hips, front of thighs, back of thighs, calves, shoulders, chest, upper back, lower back, abdominals, front of upper arms, back of upper arms) following the intensity and time recommendations in this chapter. Remember to modify some of the strength exercises to help improve your balance.

The advanced program prescribes aerobic activity five days a week and strength-building exercises on three days. Alternatively, you can do strength-building exercises on six days by exercising muscles of the upper body every other day (shoulders, chest, back, arms) and muscles of the lower body (hips, thighs, calves, abdominals) on alternate days.

You should do flexibility exercises (stretches) for all major muscle groups as part of the cool-down at the end of the session after doing aerobic and strength-building exercises. Choose stretches for the hips, legs, calves, shoulders, back, chest, and arms. Although the muscles within the ankles, wrists, and fingers are small, don't forget to stretch them.

Lifestyle physical activity every day or nearly every day should be the foundation of both programs. Sports, recreational activities, and leisure activities can be included or substituted to add variety.

Table 10.3 Model Programs for Balanced Fitness

Day of the week	Beginning program	Advanced program	Alternative advanced program
Sunday	Lifestyle physical activity	Aerobic activity Stretching Lifestyle physical activity	Aerobic activity Stretching Lifestyle physical activity
Monday	Aerobic activity Stretching Lifestyle physical activity	Aerobic activity Stretching Lifestyle physical activity	Aerobic activity Stretching Strength building and balance—lower body Lifestyle physical activity
Tuesday	Strength building Stretching Lifestyle physical activity	Strength building Stretching Lifestyle physical activity	Aerobic activity Stretching Strength building—upper body Lifestyle physical activity
Wednesday	Aerobic activity Stretching Lifestyle physical activity	Aerobic activity Stretching Lifestyle physical activity	Aerobic activity Stretching Strength building and balance—lower body Lifestyle physical activity
Thursday	Strength building Stretching Lifestyle physical activity	Strength building Aerobic activity Stretching Lifestyle physical activity	Aerobic activity Stretching Strength building—upper body Lifestyle physical activity
Friday	Aerobic activity Stretching Lifestyle physical activity	Aerobic activity Stretching Lifestyle physical activity	Aerobic activity Stretching Strength building and balance—lower body Lifestyle physical activity
Saturday	Lifestyle physical activity Stretching	Strength building Stretching Lifestyle physical activity	Aerobic activity Stretching Strength building—upper body Lifestyle physical activity

Personal Profile

Linda, Age 68

Linda started a walking program about three months ago. She has worked up to doing 30 minutes of brisk walking three days per week. She has decided to expand her fitness program to include strength-building exercises and stretching. She followed our model for a balanced fitness program to develop her personal contract for physical activity. Linda continued her walking program on Mondays, Wednesdays, and Fridays, adding stretches during her cool-down period. On Tuesdays and Thursday, she performed strength-building exercises using handheld weights or body weight activities. She included a different group of stretches on these days. Linda tried to include lifestyle physical activities every day of the week—doing household chores and walking to do errands. On weekends, instead of structured exercise, she enjoyed recreational activities or playing with her grandchildren. Linda says that the variety and her personal contract helped her stay motivated.

Summary

Now you know about all the important components of a balanced fitness program for people over age 50—aerobics, strength building, balance, and flexibility. You also know how to use the FITT program to develop your individualized program. You will never be at a loss for variety if you include all these types of exercise.

Always keep in mind the benefits of physical activity that are most important to you. If you have to stop exercising for more than a few weeks, cut back your effort to about half your previous level when you resume activity.

Chapter Checklist

Following are some ways in which you can apply what you have learned in this chapter to your daily life. Over the next few days and weeks try to do as many of these activities as possible. If you're struggling to become or stay active, you will find the review of skills in this checklist helpful.

❑ Decide which strength-building equipment you prefer to use (handheld weights, resistance rubber bands, weight machines). Of course, you can use a combination of methods if you prefer. You may need to start with the resistance provided by your body weight. You can always use equipment for resistance later.

❑ Review the strength-building and balance exercises and the stretches illustrated in this chapter. Pick one strength and balance exercise for each major muscle group. Pick one stretch for each muscle group.

❏ Use the model program for balanced fitness to plan a program to meet your needs. Write exactly what you will do each day on a personal contract for exercise.

❏ Write exactly what you will do each day on a personal contract for exercise. Keep a log of all the physical activity you do and review it regularly.

Revisit earlier skills as needed:

❏ Are you having trouble setting aside time for physical activity? See chapter 4.

❏ Are you not sure what type of physical activity to do? See chapters 6 and 7.

❏ Are others sabotaging your efforts to stay active? See chapter 8.

❏ Have you lost focus in your quest to become more active? See the information on setting goals and rewarding yourself in chapter 5.

❏ Are you becoming bored with your physical activity routine? See chapters 9 and 10.

Word Search

See if you can find 10 important words from this chapter in the grid that follows. Words appear forward and backward in rows, columns, and diagonals. The solution is shown on page 232.

```
D R I U L A T J N R Q K A R S
Y O P W E R E V E Q V X S U E
J T G Q A C P S G F W Q T B T
G O R U N V I T K X V B X B S
D L J A A S I K Y L C G G E A
Y L L H T X D O S X X W J R L
M A E A T H G I E W Y D O B N
B M N H E K Z A N S H E P A O
O C V R D K Z Z I U P H L N Q
E X E P P N C A H B E O R D K
S P U F W K A W C B S E R S W
S T R E T C H H A E E I Y T T
F F Q U D V W Z M Y G G E R S
M O N Z O N L D V W I B P M A
R W B Z V P U G U U L F R E L
```

Balance	Reps	Sets
Body weight	Resistance	Sports
Handheld	Rubber bands	Stretch
Machines		

Learn From Lapses and Manage Stress

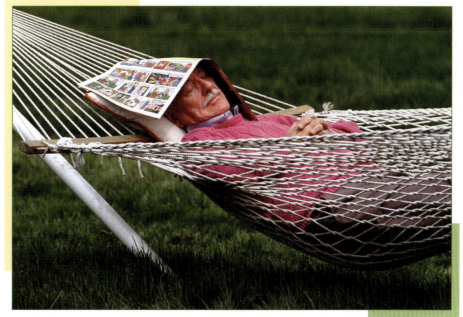

In This Chapter

❏ Assess your confidence to stay active in difficult situations.

❏ Review some of the common causes of lapses for people over age 50.

❏ Evaluate a lapse as a learning opportunity.

❏ Learn ways to get back on track quickly.

❏ Know how to prevent lapses in the future.

❏ Use physical activity to manage stress.

The objective of *Fitness After 50* is to help you learn skills to stay active for the rest of your life. But everyone who starts an activity program will have difficulty staying with it at some time or another. Avoiding setbacks and getting back on track are lifelong challenges. We would be remiss if we didn't give appropriate attention to the common problem of dealing with and preventing lapses.

Research News You Can Use

The question: How common are lapses and relapses?

The answer: A study of 7,135 YMCA members reported that 81 percent of them had at least one lapse during the year. For this study, a lapse was defined as not going to the YMCA for at least seven days in a row. The average number of lapses per member was 4.8 per year. The average length of a lapse was 36 days. Another study found that 40 percent of regular exercisers reported experiencing one or more relapses. This study defined a relapse as no exercise for at least three months (Marcus et al. 2000).

How you can use this news: Lapses in physical activity do occur. If you find that you have been inactive for at least seven days, think about what is keeping you from being active. Try to keep the length of a lapse short. Get back on track as quickly you can. Don't let a lapse turn into an excuse for not being active at all.

Having lapses in physical activity is normal. You can use lapses as learning experiences to learn what you can do to get back on track and keep from lapsing again. This chapter will show you how.

Your Confidence to Stay Active

A high level of confidence is a good predictor of doing well in the future. Your confidence level may even be a better predictor than how you did in the past. In other words, if you think you can stay active, then it's likely that you will. A research study found that general feelings of confidence and confidence related to staying active played different roles in starting and staying with physical activity. Feeling confident about physical activity was most important when first adopting new habits. General feelings of confidence were most important for people who had been active for a longer period (McAuley 1992).

Complete action box 11.1 to identify times that may be a problem for you. Refer to the tips to help you deal with many of these problems.

Action Box 11.1: How Confident Are You?

Listed here are some times when you may be tempted to stop being active. Add others to the list that are likely to be problems for you. Use the confidence scale to rate how confident you are that you can stay active. Develop a plan for any situation in which your confidence score is below 50. If the situation is not a potential problem for you, write "NA" (not applicable) in the space for the score. People who have been active regularly for more than six months (the maintenance stage of the stages of change) typically score high on most of these items.

CONFIDENCE SCALE		
NOT CONFIDENT AT ALL	**SOMEWHAT CONFIDENT**	**VERY CONFIDENT**
0 10 20 30	40 50 60 70	80 90 100
Times when you might be tempted to stop being active		**Confidence score**
Your partner didn't show up.		
Your spouse is sick.		
The weather is extremely cold, or it is hot and humid.		
The pollen count is high, and you have allergies.		
It's raining.		
You've sprained your ankle and will be on crutches for a week.		
You must travel out of town on business.		
You're feeling blue.		
You stayed up too late and overslept.		
Your workout clothes are dirty.		
You had major surgery.		
You're bored with the activity you are doing.		
You've been inactive for five days.		
You've been inactive for two weeks.		
You've gained some weight.		
You want to watch a miniseries on television.		
You're going to lots of holiday parties.		
The fitness equipment (bike, treadmill) that you typically use is broken.		

Ways to Stay Active

You will undoubtedly run into some obstacles that cause you to miss being physically active for a time. Let's look at some common barriers and some actions you can take to overcome them.

If You Get Hurt

The only way to guarantee that you will never have an injury is never to be active. Although you can't plan for injuries, expect a few minor discomforts from time to time. Here are ways to stay active if you get hurt.

■ If you twist, sprain, or strain a joint or limb, follow the four steps (RICE) for treating minor injuries. You can also use acetaminophen, ibuprofen, aspirin, or other mild, over-the-counter pain medications. Resume your physical activity as the injury or pain improves.

■ Reduce the intensity of your original activity and see whether your injury heals.

■ Look for another activity that doesn't stress the injured part. If you cannot perform your golf swing because of low back pain or if your elbow gives you trouble when you play tennis, consider walking in your neighborhood or around a park. Try walking, cycling, strength training with light weights, or swimming.

■ Modify the activity to protect the injured part. For example, if you swim and develop shoulder bursitis, use only your legs and feet for propulsion, perhaps using swim fins and a kickboard.

■ Continue to set aside time for physical activity. Once you find time for physical activity, protect it even if you get injured.

If You Get Sick

Illness can disrupt your activity program. The illness may be as minor as a sore throat or as major as a heart attack or stroke. How sick must you be before you stop your physical activity? Hard-and-fast rules are few. Let common sense and some general principles be your guide. Specific advice on physical activity for people with special health problems appears in chapter 3.

■ Always listen to your body. If you have a stuffy head from a cold and no fever, gentle physical activity may make you feel better. But if you take a walk when you have a mild cold and feel very tired or much worse after you have walked for a few minutes, stop and return home. Stay with light activity until you're feeling better and then gradually return to your previous level of activity.

RICE Method for Treating Minor Injuries

R—rest: Rest the part of the body that was injured. The amount of rest that you'll need will vary with the severity of the injury. With most minor injuries you can safely continue physical activity at lower intensity. You may improve faster by moving around some rather than resorting to complete rest.

I—ice: As soon as possible after the injury, apply ice to the area. Cold reduces swelling, bleeding, inflammation, and pain. But don't apply ice directly to your skin. Wrap the ice or ice pack with a cloth. A general rule is to apply the ice for 20 to 30 minutes and then remove it for at least 30 minutes. You can repeat the process three times a day.

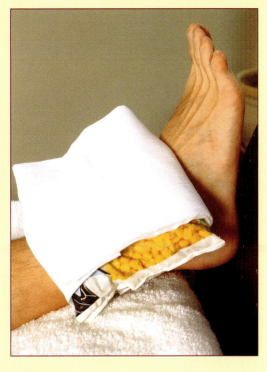

Grab a pack of frozen vegetables from the freezer for a quick, easy ice pack.

C—compression: Gentle pressure applied along with ice helps reduce swelling. Apply compression with an elastic bandage. When applying the bandage, use consistent, even pressure. Don't wrap the bandage so tightly that it reduces the blood flow. If the swelling is severe, loosen the wrap every half hour and then reapply it.

E—elevation: At first, elevate the injured part above the level of your heart, even while sleeping, until the swelling decreases. Gravity prevents the pooling of blood and other fluids, improves blood flow, and helps reduce swelling.

■ Never do physical activity or exercise when you have a fever or pain and symptoms below the neck, such as muscular pain from the flu. Your body needs to direct its energy to fighting the illness and to repairing itself. You should be free of fever for at least 48 hours before returning to physical activity. Gradually return to your previous level of activity as your strength and stamina improve. Use the skills and repeat the steps that helped you get started when you first began to increase your physical activity.

■ Never ignore pain, pressure, or a sense of fullness in your chest that occurs with physical activity. Be especially alert to pain or pressure coming from the jaw, shoulder, or arm. See table 1.4 on page 13 for normal and abnormal symptoms during physical activity. If you notice abnormal symptoms when you are physically active, especially if they go away when you stop and rest, call your doctor immediately.

■ Don't expect to go back immediately to doing the same amount of activity that you were doing before your illness. If your illness forced you to be inactive for several days or longer, you will have lost some fitness. The longer you were inactive, the more fitness you will have lost. You will need to reduce your activity program when you start again. Keep a positive attitude and don't get discouraged. With confidence and good dedication to your activity goals, you can start again. With a little time, you'll be back at the same, or a better, fitness level.

Myth Busters

Myth: Heart attack is a man's disease.

Fact: Men are indeed more likely than women to have heart attacks before age 50. Doctors believe that the female hormone estrogen protects women against heart attacks until menopause. But after menopause, a woman's risk of heart attack begins to rise. By age 65, a woman's risk of having a heart attack is about equal to that of a man. Overall, heart disease is the number one killer of women in most parts of the world. In the United States, heart disease claims six times as many lives as breast cancer does. Women are twice as likely as men are to die following a heart attack or to have a second, fatal heart attack. This disparity occurs because warning signs are often missed or misdiagnosed. Women should not fool themselves into thinking that they can't have a heart attack.

Personal Profile

Frank, Age 69

Frank's regular physical activity program is walking for 45 minutes in his neighborhood. He's been doing it every day or nearly every day for years. Unfortunately, Frank developed pneumonia and was hospitalized for five days. Even in the hospital, the nurses insisted that he get up every day for a few minutes. When he was released to go home, he made an effort to get up and move around the house every day, doing some daily activities. His wife worked, so he prepared his lunch, walked to the mailbox for the mail, and did the laundry. After two weeks, he resumed walking for 10 minutes at a time at a slow pace. The first day, he had to stop and rest after only 5 minutes. But gradually he was able to increase the length of his walks. Frank needed about two months before he could walk the full 45 minutes at one time. He's glad to have his strength and stamina back and be enjoying his regular routine.

Myth Buster

Myth: Doctors recommend bed rest and inactivity after illnesses and surgeries.

Fact: That approach has been proved wrong. In many cases, bed rest can delay recovery of previous level of physical activity. Starting light activities, such as getting out of bed and walking to the bathroom, as soon as possible is an important part of the healing process. Light activities are typically recommended even after major surgery. Always talk with your doctor about what types and levels of physical activity are possible after an illness or after surgery. Certain types of physical activity may interfere with the healing of an incision.

If Family Responsibilities Interfere With Activity

At some time, family responsibilities will interfere with your activity program. Family responsibilities differ with life stages. You will likely have family responsibilities even as you get older.

- Don't neglect your family responsibilities in favor of your physical activity program. Remember, however, that taking care of yourself is important. You can't support or care for others if you neglect your needs.

- Protect some time for yourself.

- Ask for help from other family members if you need it.

- Seek professional help or support from community agencies.

- Invite your spouse or partner to join you for activity. Being active together can be one of your best times for communication. If you walk together, you can listen without distractions to your partner's news or daily concerns. You may need to cut back on the intensity of your activity if your partner is just getting started.

If Social Activities Keep You From Being Active

When you have leisure time, you probably want to spend it with friends. Perhaps you like to go with your friends to concerts or ball games, or play bridge. These activities are stimulating and enjoyable, but they don't provide much physical activity. Consider these ways to stay active:

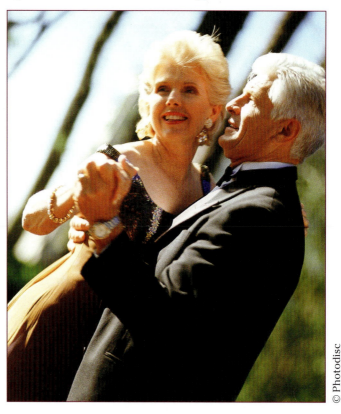

Combine social activities with physical activity, such as dancing.

- Look for more active recreation that you and your friends can enjoy together. Dancing, hiking, bicycle riding, bird watching, golfing, fishing, and traditional sports all offer good ways to combine social activities with physical activity. You will also make new friends who value physical activity.

- Let your friends know that you are concerned about being too inactive and that you are trying to become more physically active. You may be surprised at how many of them will want to join you in your effort to be more active.

- Don't ignore friends or give up activities that you enjoy to be physically active. At the same time, don't let your inactive friends sabotage your efforts to be active.

If Work Interferes With Activity

Your work or volunteer commitments may prevent you from being active. When they do, keep these alternatives in mind.

- Do your activity before going to work. People who are active first thing in the morning before dressing for the day are the most regular. Most unexpected interruptions come at the end of the day rather than at the beginning. By being active in the morning, the activity is done and over with. You feel energized and prepared to face the day.

- Try to fit brief, unscheduled periods of activity into your daily routine. Try taking a five-minute walk every two or three hours. Perhaps you can go around the block, climb a flight of stairs in your building, or simply take a brisk walk down the hall and back. Taking this short amount of time away from your work will not make you less productive. In fact, you will likely feel better and concentrate better after a brief activity break.

■ Relieve inactive work habits by building activity into the job. Find a park near your office and meet with coworkers to take a brisk 15- to 20-minute walk through the park. If you manage projects or supervise others, walk to their offices and workstations.

If You Must Travel

Travel, either for business or for pleasure, offers many possibilities for increasing your physical activity. Here are just a few:

■ Make reservations at hotels that have fitness centers or pools. Many moderately priced hotels have small fitness rooms with a few cardio-vascular machines. Some have televisions so that you can catch up on the news of the day while being active.

■ Carry your walking shoes with you, check your luggage or stow it in a locker, and take a brisk walk through the airport terminal while waiting for your plane.

■ Inquire at your hotel about a nearby park or trail. Some hotels provide maps of areas for walking or jogging. Take a brisk walk in the morning before breakfast. Nothing can energize you more or better prepare you for the events of the day like activity early in the morning.

■ Walk rather than take a taxi to your appointments. Look for time during the day to build in a few minutes of physical activity. A short walk before or after lunch will heighten your senses and make you more productive the rest of the day.

■ Try some activity at the end of a day of meetings. Go for a walk before going to your room or out to dinner. You'll feel much better.

If You Are on Vacation or Holiday

For many older adults, the desire to travel after retirement is a strong motivator to stay with an activity program. You can't enjoy traveling to the fullest if you have poor stamina or physical problems caused by inactivity. Following are some ways to stay active, avoiding a lapse, while you are on holiday.

■ Try a recreational activity that you have not tried before.

■ Explore the sights and sounds by walking. Many popular cities offer walking tours.

- Walk to parks and museums. Avoid taking the tourist bus. Why ride when you can walk?

- Plan to spend part of your time enjoying walking and biking paths. Many cities, like Sydney, San Francisco, Chicago, and Ottawa, have waterfronts on rivers, oceans, or lakes where you can walk or even bike.

- Take an ecotourism vacation. Find one with an activity that you enjoy. Fishing, hunting, bird watching, horseback riding, canoeing, cross-country skiing, and bicycling keep you active while you take a break from your normal routine.

- Be active on cruises. Cruises are known to be culinary experiences. If you don't want to arrive home with extra weight that is more than souvenirs, be active. Walk on the deck, use the fitness

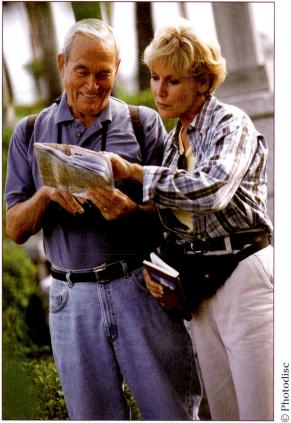

Be active so that you can enjoy traveling during your retirement.

center, take the stairs instead of the elevator, or take dance lessons. Look for day trips that include activity, such as snorkeling, hiking, cycling, or kayaking. Save the cost of the taxi or bus tour and see the area on foot. Even shopping for souvenirs counts as physical activity.

Do You Know?

If your travels take you to higher elevations, be aware of altitude sickness. How people adjust to increases in altitude varies greatly, even among those who are extremely fit. If you have cardiac and pulmonary diseases, altitudes over 5,000 feet (1,500 meters) can cause serious problems. Initial symptoms of altitude sickness include

- shortness of breath,

- headaches,

- dizziness,

- nausea, and

- difficulty sleeping.

If you experience severe shortness of breath, return to lower altitudes as soon as possible. If symptoms don't go away, get medical help. Usually, minor symptoms of breathlessness disappear within a day or two. To prevent altitude sickness while you adjust to higher elevations, reduce the intensity of your activity, get adequate rest, and avoid alcohol.

High-Risk Situations

You can learn to manage high-risk situations, which are times when you may be inactive. Thinking and planning ahead are crucial. Try to identify in advance when you'll face situations that encourage inactivity. Look back at your confidence scores from earlier in this chapter. Come up with several ways in which you could stay active. After you have experienced a high-risk situation, evaluate how you handled it using action box 11.2. Several examples show how others have managed situations that interfered with their physical activity plans.

Action Box 11.2: Evaluating High-Risk Situations

Describe what happened in a high-risk situation within the last few weeks.

Before the situation? _____

During the situation? _____

After the situation? _____

Overall, how well did you handle the situation? Rate your success on a scale of 1 to 5.

Not very well				Very well
1	2	3	4	5

If you believe that you were successful (rating of 3 or higher), what was the key to your success? _____

If you believe that you were unsuccessful (rating below 3), what could you do differently next time? _____

(continued)

➠**Action Box 11.2: Evaluating High-Risk Situations** *(continued)*

Before the situation? _____

_____

During the situation? _____

_____

After the situation? _____

_____

_____

Personal Profile

Jim, Age 58

Before the situation? Jim had worked late the night before at the office and gotten home late. He had a lot on his mind, so he had a difficult time getting to sleep. He woke up several times during the night worrying about what to do with problems at work. Because he typically exercises in the mornings, he packed his workout bag and laid out his clothes for work.

During the situation? When the alarm went off at 6:00 a.m., he was feeling extremely tired and was tempted to hit the snooze button and sleep in for an hour instead of getting up to exercise. He remembered that his workout bag was ready to go. He really had no good reason to miss the exercise session. Jim knew that exercise would likely reenergize him and help him feel prepared to handle another day that was also likely to be stressful. He recognized that he could use the time riding the stationary cycle to develop new problem-solving strategies. He turned off the alarm and slowly got out of bed. Within a few minutes, he was headed for the health club.

After the situation? Jim did his usual morning exercise and felt good about it. He not only felt reenergized but also felt in control of his actions and confident about the work-related issues that had been on his mind. In addition, he made a commitment to practice relaxation techniques to help him get to sleep when faced with a night like the one before. Overall, he rated his success in handling this situation as a 4+.

Jim's key to success was his management of cues. Because the workout bag was ready to go, he followed his usual routine, even though he felt tired. If he had forgotten to pack the bag, he may well have decided to sleep in. He also changed from thinking about sleep to recognizing that he would feel energized and could use the time for problem solving.

Personal Profile

Debbie, Age 70

Before the situation? Debbie lives alone. She typically goes for a 30-minute walk in her neighborhood before dinner almost every evening. She missed walking yesterday because of rain, so she was eager to get outdoors today. Just as Debbie was about to step out the door, a friend called to ask her to go out to eat.

During the situation? Debbie didn't have anything planned or prepared for dinner and would have enjoyed a night out with her friend. She asked her friend to join her for the walk, but the friend said no and didn't want to wait because she didn't feel like being out after dark. The friend, who isn't active, suggested that it wouldn't matter if Debbie missed the walk. She could walk another time. "Isn't our friendship important to you?" she asked. Debbie didn't want to disappoint her friend, so she gave up her walk and went out to eat.

After the situation? By the time she got home, Debbie felt sluggish from overeating. She read for a while and then went to bed. Although she enjoyed the time with her friend, she was upset with herself for missing her walk. She rated her handling of the situation as a 2.

Debbie assessed the cues associated with the situation and identified several ways to handle a similar situation in the future.

Before the situation? Debbie could look for ways to include as much lifestyle activity as possible in her daily routines. If she is getting short bouts of activity throughout the day, then she doesn't feel so bad if something comes up to cause her to miss her walk. In addition, Debbie could find an alternative place to walk when the weather is poor, such as a shopping mall. Debbie could rehearse ways to respond to others who make requests or use statements that sabotage her goals. If Debbie does not have any friends who are active, she could try to make new friends who share her active lifestyle. (You should avoid the naysayers and surround yourself with people who share your values when you are trying to adopt new habits.)

During the situation? Debbie could say, "Of course, your friendship is important to me, but being active is important to me too. I'll go with you this time, but in the future, please give me more notice so I can walk before we go out." Alternatively, she could say, "Of course, your friendship is important to me, but being active is important to me too. Thanks for the invitation, but this time I must say no. Let's plan another time that works for both of us."

After the situation? If Debbie agrees to the request, she should feel good about her decision, set boundaries for what she will eat and drink, plan another

(continued)

time to be active, and enjoy the evening. Would it be too late to work out with a stretching video before bedtime? If Debbie refuses the request, she should enjoy her walk. In a few days, she could invite her friend to go for a walk or on some other outing that involves physical activity, perhaps shopping at a flea market or visiting a museum.

Getting Back on Track Quickly

Remember the stages of change process introduced earlier in this book? Recall that change is not linear. People don't march in a forward, stepwise fashion from one stage of change to the next. The expression "two steps forward and one step back" is an accurate description of how change occurs. Such patterns are normal and natural. Ideally, if you lapse (and you will!), you will go only one step back in the change process.

Complete the Readiness to Change Questionnaire one more time (see pages 2 and 3 in chapter 1). What stage are you in?

The more quickly you can move back into the action stage, the more likely it is that you'll succeed at reestablishing and maintaining physical activity for a lifetime. Most people will cycle through the stages of change several times before getting to the maintenance stage for good. Don't let lapsing back to a previous stage make you feel embarrassed or guilty. Don't apply negative labels to yourself ("slug," "dumb," "couch potato") after a lapse. Negative self-talk could cause you to lapse more than one stage.

Fortunately, most people don't go all the way back to the precontemplation stage (not thinking about being active at all) after a lapse. Your position in the stage of change process may give you an idea of how quickly you'll be able to get back to regular physical activity after a lapse:

■ You will probably return to regular activity quickly if you have made several serious attempts to change in the past. The more often you have made a serious attempt in the past, the better your chance of long-term success on your next attempt. The key is learning from the lapse and trying something different on the next attempt.

■ You are likely to resume regular physical activity if you are in a later stage of change when the lapse occurs. People who are in the maintenance stage have the least difficulty with lapses, even lapses for long periods. They know and value the benefits of being active and have the confidence and skills to get back on track as soon as whatever caused the lapse is no longer a problem. People who are in the action stage are at a high risk for lapses but can usually get back on track quickly if they don't allow too much time to pass before starting again.

■ Resumption of regular physical activity is more likely if you can progress from one stage to the next within about one month. For example, suppose that someone who was in the preparation stage stops moving forward with plans to be active and returns to just thinking about activity (contemplation stage). If he or she can progress within a month from thinking about being active again to going for a walk every now and then, the chance for success is good. The person who needs more than a month to get back on track can easily become stuck in the contemplation stage.

■ You will probably return to regular activity quickly if you are using the processes and skills appropriate for your stage of change.

Use the tips for getting back on track in action box 11.3. If necessary, use the Readiness to Change Questionnaire in the appendix to determine your stage when your lapse occurred.

Action Box 11.3: Getting Back on Track

Use these tips to help you get back to activity after a lapse for specific stages of change. If you experience a lapse, select a tip for your stage and try it. If you have experienced lapses in the past, mark the tips that have worked for you. They are likely to work again. Add other ideas in the space provided.

PRECONTEMPLATION AND CONTEMPLATION STAGES:
Not thinking about being active or thinking about
becoming active, but not yet doing any activity

- Consider whether you are embracing or resisting the goal of being physically active.
- Identify and focus on the benefits (pros) of physical activity that are important to you.
- Read or learn something new about physical activity.
- Think about the warnings of the health hazards of inactivity.
- Remind yourself that you are the only one who is responsible for your health and well-being.
- Talk to people like yourself who are physically active.
- Think of ways to substitute physical activity for times when you are inactive.
- Identify your barriers to being active (your cons).
- Visualize yourself as an active person.
- Reward yourself for thinking about being active again.

PREPARATION STAGE:
Doing some activity from time to time, but not regularly

- Think about how confident you will feel if you start to be active again.
- Tell yourself that you want to be active. Use affirmations to build your confidence.
- Make a new commitment to be active and start again.
- Believe that regular physical activity will make you a healthier, happier person.
- Make a personal contract to be active again. Set small goals and reward yourself for making progress.
- Be sure that you have a convenient place to be active.
- Arrange your surroundings to support your activity. Give yourself cues to be active.

(continued)

➡**Action Box 11.3: Getting Back on Track** *(continued)*

PREPARATION STAGE: **Doing some activity from time to time, but not regularly *(continued)***

- Keep records of the activity that you do and check your progress.
- Develop a balanced fitness program that includes aerobic, strength, balance, and flexibility exercises.
- Schedule time for physical activity and make it a priority.
- Start again slowly. Commit to being active for at least 15 minutes each day.
- Plan for high-risk situations that might keep you from being active.
- Ask someone to support you in your effort to increase your activity.
- Think of ways to make physical activity fun.
- Reward yourself for getting started again.

ACTION STAGE: **Active regularly, but not long enough for activity to become a habit**

- Remind yourself that being active is part of your personal value system.
- Set realistic goals for yourself. Don't expect to start back at your previous activity level.
- Keep records of the activity that you do. Give yourself time to build up your fitness level.
- Identify someone who will encourage you to be active when you don't feel up to it.
- Have someone provide feedback to you about your physical activity.
- Keep objects around your home and workplace that remind you to be active.
- Remove obstacles from your surroundings that contribute to your inactivity.
- Avoid spending long periods in settings that encourage inactivity.
- Do some physical activity, even when you feel tired. You know that you will feel better afterward.
- Use activity to relieve your worries when you are feeling tense.
- If boredom is a problem, try a new physical activity that you have not done recently.
- Remind yourself that you have been active before and that you can be active again.

Research News You Can Use

Question: Who is an exercise dropout?

Answer: People's thoughts about whether they had dropped out of exercise were related to the amount of time since they stopped exercising and to their previous exercise experience (Dubbert and Stetson 1995). Those who had been exercising regularly for the longest time before their lapse reported longer periods of inactivity before thinking of themselves as having dropped out.

How you can use this news: Continue to think of yourself as an active person even when your activity has been interrupted. Visualize the time when you were active. Use affirmations to tell yourself that you will be active again. Feel confident that even if your activity is interrupted for weeks or months, you can start again.

Prevent Lapses in the Future

When you are headed toward a lapse, you are likely to reach several points where you can change your actions to prevent the lapse. Two scenarios are described in action box 11.4. What would you do in these situations? Remember that you can change your thoughts and feelings as well as your actions.

Action Box 11.4: Stop the Chain of Events

Can you think of other ways in which you might have prevented these lapses? Add your ideas in the space provided.

Chain of events	Preventive strategy
Monday—It rains so you can't walk outdoors.	Climb stairs in your office building. Vacuum the carpet at home, working as fast as you can to burn more calories.
Tuesday—The rain continues. You miss another day of activity.	Drive to a shopping mall to walk. Work out with a fitness video in your home.
Wednesday—You must go out of town on a trip. You spend most of your time in the airport.	Make reservations at a hotel with a fitness center or swimming pool. Store or check your luggage and walk in the airport while waiting for your flight.
Thursday—The people you are with are mostly inactive.	Tell yourself that this trip will not cause you to stop your activity altogether. Get up early and work out in the fitness center at the hotel.
Friday—When you return home, you feel too tired to do anything.	Do something active even if you don't feel like it. Physical activity relieves fatigue and helps you sleep better. Ask your spouse or a friend to remind you to be active.
Saturday and Sunday—Because you've been out of town all week, you want to spend time with your family. You realize that it has been a week since you participated in any activity.	Get up early and go for a walk by yourself. Enjoy the quiet time after a hectic week. Plan an activity that the family can do together—biking, hiking, or skating. Resolve to resume your regular program on Monday.

Physical Activity for Stress Management

Physical activity has been called nature's own tranquilizer because of its calming effect on the body and mind. Physical activity also makes your vital organs (heart, lungs, blood vessels) stronger and better able to function properly when faced with stress. Your body will become stress hardy because of regular physical activity and exercise.

People who are physically active say that they sleep better at night. Rather than feeling tired, however, most people say that they feel reenergized after activity. Regular physical activity is a valid stress management technique.

Stress Management Tips

Follow these tips when using physical activity to manage your stress:

- If you are the aggressive type, avoid competitive physical activity for stress management purposes. You might overexert yourself.

- If you are facing a tense situation or doing a tedious task, take a break and go for a walk. Getting away for a few minutes helps you clear your mind and view problems in a new way.

- If your day is often hectic, plan physical activity at the end of the day to rid the body of harmful stress by-products that have built up during the day.

Personal Profile

Margaret, Age 53

Margaret, an elementary school teacher, is beginning to experience some of the physical and emotional changes of menopause. The worst symptom is night sweats, which interrupt her sleep. Margaret finds that on the days when she is more physically active, she sleeps better. The hot flashes haven't gone away, but she is able to get back to sleep more quickly and feels rested the next day. Physical activity also raises her spirits and makes her feel youthful.

Relaxation Techniques

Everyone feels tense from time to time. When you do, practice one of these relaxation techniques. Use action box 11.5 to develop a plan for learning to relax. As with any new habit, you must practice these techniques to get a benefit.

- Deep-breathing exercises—You've heard this before: Take a deep breath and relax. Taking more than one deep breath is even better. Begin by breathing in slowly and deeply through your nose. While breathing in, count to five and silently say the word "in" to yourself. Notice that your abdomen relaxes as your lungs fill with air. After the count of five, slowly let the air out as you count to five and say the word "out" to yourself. Repeat the exercise for at least five minutes. You may do these exercises while sitting, standing, or lying down. For best results, get comfortable by loosening your tie, belt, or buttons. A quiet place is recommended, but not necessary. Deep breathing is the first step of many relaxation techniques, so practice and learn to do it anywhere.

- Visualization—Begin with a few minutes of deep breathing. Then close your eyes and create a mental image of a scene in which you are perfectly relaxed. Imagine that you are walking in a rain forest, sailing on a boat in the ocean, or overlooking over a beautiful valley from the top of a mountain. Continue to breathe deeply. Involve all your senses in escaping to your special place. What sounds do you hear? How does the air smell and feel on your skin? Are you feeling as relaxed as if you were really there? Visualization gives your mind a rest when you are feeling stressed. Many people say that some of their most creative ideas and solutions come after visualizations.

- Progressive muscle relaxation—At first, you should do this technique while lying down. Choose a quiet place where you will not be disturbed for at least 20 minutes. Begin with deep-breathing exercises. Try to relax your entire body. Starting at your feet and working up your body, contract each muscle group tightly as you inhale. Hold the contraction for a few seconds; then exhale and relax. Let the tension flow out with each breath. Notice the feel of the muscles as they contract and relax. Move up the body from the feet to the calves, thighs, buttocks, abdomen, hands, arms, and shoulders. End with the muscles of the face, mouth, jaw, eyes, and scalp. Allow more time for the relaxation phase of the exercise. If a muscle seems particularly tense, repeat the contraction for that muscle group. When you finish, lie very still for at least five minutes. (You may want to include a visualization exercise at this time.) When you are ready to get up, count backward from 10 to 1. Get up slowly and carefully. Do progressive muscle relaxation daily for best results. With practice, you can learn to do progressive muscle relaxation while sitting in a chair.

- Stretching—Most people hold tension in their head, neck, and shoulder areas (called the stress triangle). The base of the triangle is the midpoint between your shoulders and neck. The top of the triangle is on your forehead between your eyes. Stretching can help relieve tension in your stress triangle. Stop and do a few stretches, especially when you are doing a tedious task. More about stretching is provided in chapter 10.

  Overhead stretch—With one arm, reach up as if you were reaching for an object on a high shelf. Repeat with the other arm.

Shoulder shrugs—Lift your shoulders up and make large circles going forward and backward. You can rotate both shoulders or stretch one at a time.

Neck roll—Keep your left shoulder level while stretching the right ear to the right shoulder. Roll your head down so that your chin is on your chest. Repeat the stretch with your left side. Do not let your head drop back.

■ Self-massage—You can learn to give yourself a massage. Massage relaxes muscles, relieves pain, increases blood flow to the skin and muscles, eases mental stress, and helps you feel more relaxed.

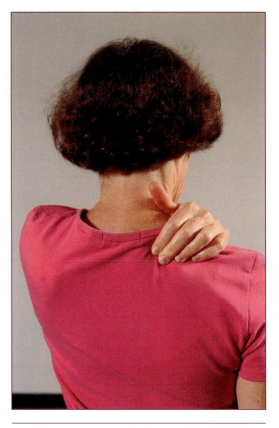

Give yourself a massage to relax muscles and ease mental stress.

Shoulder and back of neck—Massage your stress triangle, using your left hand to work on your right shoulder and your right hand to work on your left shoulder. Begin at your shoulder blade and move up toward the back of your neck, including the scalp. Use a circular motion to massage the thickest part of the muscle. Repeat several times on both sides. Some health and wellness stores sell a device called a back buddy, an S-shaped item made of tubular plastic with a few knobs on it. You can use it to apply pressure to your neck and back and work on the areas where muscles feel tight.

Head and face—Use your fingers to apply pressure on your forehead between your eyes (the top point of your stress triangle). Use your thumbs to apply gentle pressure on the areas below your brow bone close to your nose. Use gentle circular motions to rub the area of your temples and behind your ears. Rub your scalp with a gentle and rapid motion as though you are shampooing your hair.

Feet—Use your thumbs to rub the full length of your foot, from the heel to the toes and back. Rub each toe individually. Hold your ankle in one hand and your toes in the other. Rotate your foot at the ankle in both directions.

Massage is not a substitute for medical treatment for an injury. See your doctor if you have an injury, such as a sprain, tendinitis, or a swollen joint.

Action Box 11.5: My Plan to Practice Relaxation

Select a relaxation technique and commit to practicing it for at least one week. Evaluate your experience.

During the week of _____, I will practice _____

_____

for at least _____ minutes per day.

Day	Minutes	Comments
Sunday		
Monday		
Tuesday		
Wednesday		
Thursday		
Friday		
Saturday		
Did you feel more relaxed?		

Summary

Lapses and setbacks occur for many reasons—some are within your control and others are not. You can usually anticipate and prepare for social activities, travel, and routine tasks. Others events, such as injuries, illnesses, special projects, and unexpected family responsibilities, may not be within your control, but you can still manage them. Your goal is not to let a lapse become a reason to give up being active entirely.

Several days, or even a few weeks, without physical activity or exercise is not a tragedy. You can regain your fitness relatively quickly once you start again if you don't wait too long. Use the skills that you have learned and applied in becoming active to get back on track.

Fortunately, most people who lapse will return to a point where they think about being active and make new plans to start again. If you view a lapse as a learning opportunity, you can evaluate it, learn from it, and begin to consider plans to start again. If you try something different the next time around, your confidence for handling high-risk situations and maintaining your physical activity will increase.

Always keep these points in mind as you move forward to try again:

- Try again as quickly as possible.
- Try again. This time you're probably at least one stage ahead of where you started last time.

- Try again but do something differently. Learn from your experience.
- Try again. You can do it!

Chapter Checklist

Following are some ways in which you can apply what you have learned in this chapter to your daily life. Over the next few days and weeks try to do as many of these activities as possible.

❑ Identify your high-risk situations. Develop a plan to handle any situation in which your confidence level score is below 50.

❑ Evaluate any lapse that you have. Turn a lapse into a learning opportunity so that you can manage similar high-risk situations in the future.

❑ If you lapse, complete the Readiness to Change Questionnaire to see where you are. Use the tips for getting back on track that are appropriate for your stage of change.

❑ Learn relaxation techniques to help relieve stress. Feeling stressed can increase your risk for a lapse.

Word Search

See if you can find 10 important words from this chapter in the grid that follows. Words appear forward and backward in rows, columns, and diagonals. The solution is shown on page 232.

```
S  G  X  T  W  C  G  H  I  E  X  D  A  F  M
S  Y  L  O  R  B  I  B  C  V  Z  F  L  M  J
E  E  M  J  H  G  G  N  V  U  W  H  T  X  E
S  G  E  P  H  R  E  L  A  X  A  T  I  O  N
P  D  A  R  T  D  D  L  M  A  F  B  T  P  I
A  U  I  S  I  O  F  V  U  B  Q  D  U  M  S
L  S  L  F  S  J  M  I  S  N  B  S  D  S  J
K  G  N  E  Z  A  J  S  R  I  C  E  E  J  R
B  O  M  E  B  H  M  L  H  A  N  R  Q  J  C
C  M  I  W  J  X  X  V  Q  X  T  P  X  Z  G
E  H  T  A  E  R  B  Q  V  S  I  Y  Q  Z  R
W  K  H  G  X  W  I  J  G  E  U  Z  R  I  C
X  Q  T  H  B  Z  H  E  F  L  K  Q  Q  A  Q
L  E  U  G  Y  T  Y  H  K  U  A  U  E  C  K
Z  P  X  D  K  P  H  Y  M  D  P  L  Y  I  M
```

Altitude	Lapses	RICE
Breathe	Massage	Stress
Confidence	Relaxation	Symptoms
High risk		

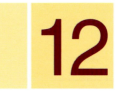

Looking Ahead

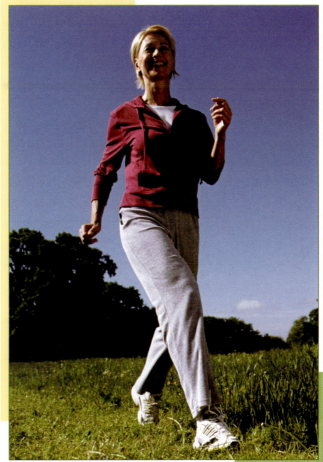

© Jumpfoto

In This Chapter

❑ Make other changes in your life.

❑ Help someone else be active.

❑ Be an advocate for physical activity in your community.

ongratulations on reaching the end of the book! We hope that this book and its approach are helping you increase your physical activity. Although you've reached the end of the book, you're not done yet. Throughout *Fitness After 50* our focus was on you and your physical activity habits. In closing, we're going to suggest some ways in which you can go beyond your own personal physical activity program to use what you have learned and practiced in *Fitness After 50*.

Making Other Changes in Your Life

You can apply the skills that you used to increase your physical activity to improve your quality of life in other ways. If you can make and sustain a change that is as important (and as difficult) as becoming and staying active, you can use what you've learned to tackle other challenges that you may face in the future.

Growing older introduces major life changes. Having an understanding of and being prepared for changes and challenges is important for maintaining quality of life. The questions that follow may help you think about some of the common challenges that most people eventually face. If you have already met some of these challenges, think about your experience and apply what you've learned to other life areas. Complete action box 12.1 to identify other changes that you need or want to make in your life.

Career Changes

- How will you spend your retirement?

- From what will you get your sense of self-worth after you retire from the workplace?

- How will you sustain social contacts with friends and colleagues when you are no longer working?

- Can you apply your talents and wisdom in new ways—a part-time job, second career, or volunteer position?

Family Changes

- Are you able to enjoy your grandchildren?

- Are you prepared to be a caregiver if a spouse or other family member is disabled by health problems?

- Will you need to move to another residence or make modifications to your home?

Personal Changes

- Can you describe the essence of who you are apart from your daily activities or the care that you provide others?

- What is your passion, and where can you find joy during this time of your life?

- Do you have issues related to forgiveness and reconciliation that you should consider?

Action Box 12.1: Other Changes I Would Like to Make

Identify aspects of your life that you would like to change. Think about why the change is important to you at this time in your life. Write a short-term goal (something you will do in the next 30 days) to get you started toward making a change.

I would like to change . . .

Because . . .

My short-term goal: _____

I would like to change . . .

Because . . .

My short-term goal: _____

I would like to change . . .

Because . . .

My short-term goal: _____

Action box 12.2 will help you identify the skills that were most helpful to you as you increased your activity level. Those that you rate very helpful are ones that you should plan to use again. You may want to review the skills that you rated as only somewhat helpful or not helpful. Some skills are more difficult and require more practice and persistence to master.

Action Box 12.2: Which Skills Did You Use?

Following is a list of the major skills introduced in this book to help you increase your physical activity level. Think back over all that you have learned and accomplished. For each skill, place a mark in the box to indicate how helpful the skill was to you. For the skills that were very helpful, make a note of how you could use them to achieve a goal in another area of your life.

Skills for making changes	Very helpful	Somewhat helpful	Not helpful
Weighing pros and cons			
Learning new information			
Seeking help and support from others			
Using rewards to reinforce positive habits			
Saying affirmations and practicing positive self-talk			
Keeping track of thoughts			
Making changes in surroundings			
Changing thoughts			
Substituting positive behaviors for negative behaviors			
Identifying triggers and cues			
Planning for high-risk situations			
Keeping records (self-monitoring)			
Setting realistic goals			
Developing a personal contract			
Managing time			
Communicating assertively			
Practicing relaxation techniques			
Solving problems			
Finding and evaluating resources			
Learning from lapses			

How I will use these skills to achieve another goal: _____

_____

_____

Influencing Others

As you become more confident about your ability to stay physically active, you may want to consider your influence on others. Just as you looked to others as positive role models when you were getting started, now you can help someone else. People who are inactive can gain no greater motivation than seeing others like themselves who have become active. They will say, "If she can do it, I can too."

Remember, however, that not everyone is ready to take action right away. Follow these tips to help an inactive friend or family member become more active.

■ Ask questions similar to those on the Readiness to Change Questionnaire to determine where your friend is in the change process. Listen to statements that he or she makes about physical activity. Review the statements of people in various stages of readiness that were listed in the introduction.

■ Share information about the numerous benefits or advantages (pros) of physical activity. Ask your friend to think about which benefits are most important to him or her at this time.

■ Answer questions honestly about your experiences when you were getting started. Don't make regular physical activity seem easy. Say that becoming active is difficult, but that it is possible and worth the effort.

■ Talk about barriers and obstacles that must be overcome to get started with physical activity. Give specific examples of how you were able to overcome your barriers and problems. Remember that lack of time is one of the most common reasons people give for being inactive. Be prepared to give specific examples of ways to fit in physical activity.

■ Brainstorm ways to replace inactive time with physical activities. If your friend is opposed to or intimidated by structured exercise, emphasize the merits of lifestyle physical activity.

■ Suggest that your friend wear your step counter for a few days to track activity. Most people are surprised at how inactive their lifestyles really are.

■ At the appropriate time, help your friend develop a plan or personal contract for activity. Sign the contract as a supporter.

■ Give appropriate praise and reinforcement along the way. Help your friend think of an appropriate reward and participate in the reward, if desired.

■ Ask about specific ways in which you can help and listen carefully to the request. Your friend is responsible for telling you what he or she wants and needs. Don't attempt to read another's mind.

■ If your friend indicates that he or she would enjoy having you as an activity partner, let the friend choose the activity and set the pace. Because of the lower intensity of your friend's program, you will probably want to continue with your more advanced program on your own. View the opportunity to be a role model as a way to increase your activity time.

Being an Advocate for Physical Activity

Our goal in writing this book was to help people become more active. We are advocates of physical activity in our professional and personal lives. If you are enjoying the benefits of physical activity, you too can be an advocate for physical activity in your community, especially for older adults.

People are living longer, as you can see from the statistics in table 12.1. The percentage of people in the over-65 age group is increasing. One of the fastest growing age groups in the world is people 85 and older.

Older adults want to see their grandchildren (and great-grandchildren) grow up. They want to be involved in their communities, and they want to live life to the fullest for as long as possible. But unless they can maintain good health, fitness, and function as they age, their quality of life will diminish and the burden they place on society will increase. The long-term benefits of physical activity are proven. The need to increase physical activity among people of all ages, especially among people age 50 and older, is critical.

Being physically active depends in part on living in communities that encourage and promote physical activity. You can help your community make it easier to walk, jog, or bike as a means of transportation as well as for lifestyle and recreational pursuits.

Table 12.1 Life Expectancy at Birth for Men and Women

	Both	Men	Women
Australia	80.3	77.4	83.3
Canada	80.0	76.6	83.5
New Zealand	78.5	75.5	81.6
United Kingdom	78.3	75.8	80.8
United States	77.4	74.6	80.4

The life expectancy in years is given for babies born in 2004.

U.S. Census Bureau; *International Data Base, Table 10—Life Expectancy at Birth by Sex: 2004.*

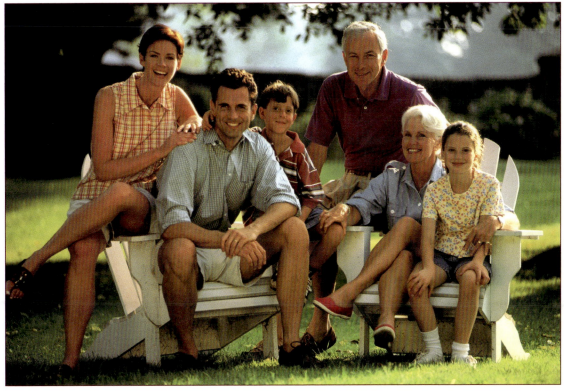

Seeing grandchildren grow into productive adults is a source of pride for many older people.

Activity-related resources in your community include everything from the air people breathe to safe sidewalks to exercise facilities. Following is a list of questions for you to ask when evaluating resources, both material and human, for physical activity in your community (USHHS 1999).

Do the physical activity resources have these features? Are they:

Available—Do resources exist? Are there places for people to be active?

Accessible—Are resources easy to get to? Are they barrier free? Are the resources available when and where they are needed?

Affordable—What are the costs involved?

Acceptable—Do people view the resource positively? Do the benefits outweigh costs?

Appropriate—Does the resource fill the need? Is the quality and quantity appropriate for the intended purpose?

Throughout this book we have discussed barriers to physical activity. As you become an advocate for physical activity, don't be surprised if you start looking at your community in a new light. Perhaps for the first time, you will find yourself paying attention to cracks in sidewalks or lights at intersection crossings. If what you find makes you question your ability to go for a walk, imagine how the person who is not yet active feels.

See the checklist in action box 12.3 to evaluate how activity friendly your community is. You can use what you find to take action. Action may mean reporting the problem to the person or department that can correct it or getting involved yourself.

Action Box 12.3: Is Your Community Activity Friendly?

Check for any barriers to physical activity that you observe in your community. Add others to the list. Make a note of the specific location so that you can take action.

Barriers to physical activity	Notes
Uneven or cracked sidewalks	
Sidewalks that are not continuous	
Narrow sidewalks with no buffers from traffic (trees, shrubs, street-side parked cars, green space)	
Unsafe street crossings	
Traffic signals that don't give pedestrians enough time to cross safely	
No bike lanes or pathways along major streets and highways	
Poorly lit streets	
Stairwells that are hard to find, dirty, poorly ventilated, and unsafe	
Lack of public transportation routes to major community parks or exercise facilities	
No markers along trails, beaches, and city blocks to help people judge distances	
No bicycle parking and storage racks at major destinations	
Buses and commuter trains without racks for carrying bikes	
Lack of signs with directions and distances to key places	
Schools that do not open their facilities to the public before and after school hours	
Outdoor playing fields without lights for evening use	
List other barriers here:	

Here are a few ideas about how you can help promote physical activity in your community for the benefit of yourself and others.

- Encourage elected officials to make community resources available to promote physical activity.

- Ask that school buildings and grounds be made available to the community at large before and after the school day, on weekends, and during holidays.

- Join community coalitions to support accessible and affordable community-based physical activity programs for the benefit of the community as a whole. Community planners and designers should consider the needs of all community members, including those with disabilities.

- Encourage employers to offer benefits that include fitness center memberships or community-based fitness classes for employees, retirees, and their families. Employers should encourage health insurers to consider lower insurance premiums for people who are physically active on a regular basis.

- Speak up at board or development meetings. Write or petition for improvements. Gather signatures. Make the media aware of problems and potential solutions.

- Organize a neighborhood speed-watch or crime-watch program.

- Encourage schools to teach pedestrian safety.

- Ask that public works departments trim trees and plants.

- Organize a community clean-up or beautification day.

- Persuade local media to do a story about the health benefits of walking.

Talk with your friends who enjoy physical activity about your ideas for making your community a more active place. Use action box 12.4 to brainstorm ideas and start to develop a plan. Contact other people and organizations in your community to build support for your ideas.

Action Box 12.4: Community Action Plan for Physical Activity Projects

The following steps can help you get started with a project. You will need to develop a more detailed plan later.

1. Identify specific needs or problems in your community. Consider short-term (one year or less) and long-term (two to five years) needs.

(continued)

➡**Action Box 12.4: Community Action Plan for Physical Activity Projects** *(continued)*

2. Brainstorm possible solutions.

3. Select one or two projects that have potential in the short term.

4. What resources are needed to support the project?

5. Who can help?

6. What action will you take immediately to get started?

Personal Profile

Advocates for Physical Activity

A group of retired friends who enjoyed walking together noticed an abandoned railroad track in their community. By exploring a little more, they learned that the track went about two miles (3 kilometers) in each direction before entering other suburban communities. They wondered whether it would be possible to convert the track into a pathway. The group organized themselves and went to work. They developed a plan and took it to the city government. Several of them contacted their former employers with businesses downtown to ask about sponsoring the project. Within a few months, hundreds of people were enjoying the pathway every day. Some are out for some activity—walking, cycling, skating. Others are walking or riding their bikes to work. Visitors to the city use the pathway to walk to museums and the theater. More remains to be done. The group would like to develop maps showing distances to points of interest along the pathway. Perhaps doctors at downtown clinics could give the maps to their patients who need to be more active. The project has received much positive publicity for the city. As a result, nearby cities want to continue the pathway through their communities. The pathway has the potential to be 40 miles (64 kilometers) long before it spills into the countryside.

We wish you all the best as you strive to stay active yourself, be an active role model for others, and be an advocate for physical activity in your community. Enjoy your journey of lifelong physical activity.

Appendix

Weigh Your Pros and Cons

Mark the pros and cons that are important to you now. For those that are very important, place two marks in the blank. Count the total number of marks in each column. Do your pros outweigh your cons?

Advantages, or pros, for physical activity	Disadvantages, or cons, for physical activity
_____ I enjoy being physically active.	_____ I'm too tired to be active.
_____ I feel better when I am active.	_____ I'm too old to be active.
_____ Being active makes me feel young.	_____ I'll appear foolish.
_____ Physical activity reduces my risk of heart attack, stroke, and even some cancers.	_____ None of my friends are active.
	_____ I could get hurt.
_____ Physical activity helps control my blood pressure, cholesterol, and triglycerides.	_____ I don't like to sweat.
	_____ My allergies prevent me from being outdoors.
_____ Being active helps prevent type 2 diabetes.	_____ I just don't like physical activity.
_____ Being active increases longevity.	_____ I wouldn't be able to do other activities that I enjoy.
_____ Staying active will help me live independently for longer.	_____ My joints hurt when I move.
_____ I can sleep better when I am active.	_____ I might have a heart attack.
_____ I am less likely to fall if I am fit.	_____ I don't have the money to join a fitness center.
_____ I like looking trim and fit.	
_____ I feel more confident and in control of my life.	_____ I don't have a safe place to be active.
	_____ I don't have the skills.
_____ Physical activity helps me manage my weight.	_____ I don't know what to do.
_____ I am able to take fewer medications.	_____ I don't want to have to leave home to do activity.
_____ My bones will be stronger if I am active.	Add your personal cons here.
_____ I will be able to do daily tasks and take care of myself.	
Add your personal pros here.	
Total for pros _____	Total for cons _____
Try to add at least one more pro to your list next week.	Try to eliminate at least one con from your list next week.

From *Fitness After 50* by W. Ettinger, B. Wright, and S. Blair, 2006, Champaign, IL: Human Kinetics.

Keep Track of Your Thoughts and Actions

Part 1: Recording Thoughts and Actions

Use this form to record the number of times that you think about doing some physical activity. Simply place a mark in a box in the left column of the table each time you *think* about doing some physical activity. If you carried out your thoughts and did the activity you were thinking about, place a mark in the right column of the table.

Day	Times that I *thought* about physical activity	Times that I *followed through* on the thought and did the physical activity
Sunday		
Monday		
Tuesday		
Wednesday		
Thursday		
Friday		
Saturday		
	Total times that I thought about physical activity: _____	Total times that I followed through on the thought: _____

Part 2: Learning From Your Thoughts

1. What triggered my thought about physical activity?

   Example: I saw a friend being active.

   _____

2. What was the thought about physical activity?

   Example: "I see that Sally is walking outside. I could do that. Maybe we can walk together." Or "I see Sally walking outside. She looks cold."

   _____

3. If your thought was negative, what could you say to yourself so that you'd be more likely to be physically active?

   Example: "As long as I wear my good coat, I'll be perfectly warm."

   _____

4. If your thought was positive, did you respond by doing some physical activity? Why or why not?

   _____

From Active Living Partners.

Personal Time Study

Make three copies of the time form. Fill in the time slots with the tasks or activities that you do over three typical days (two weekdays and one weekend day). After you've recorded your activities, determine the number of minutes that you spent doing any type of physical activity—walking, climbing stairs, gardening, housework—and your minutes of inactivity, such as sleeping, sitting, riding in a car or bus, watching television, or talking on the phone. At the bottom on the form, add up the minutes of activity (Yes column) and inactivity (No column) for the day. The total for each four-hour time slot should be 240 minutes. The total for each day should be 1,440 minutes.

Instead of (inactive times)   I will do (list activities here)

_____   _____

_____   _____

_____   _____

_____   _____

_____   _____

| | | PHYSICALLY ACTIVE? | |
Time slot	Tasks or activities	Yes	No
Midnight to 4:00 a.m.			
4:00 to 8:00 a.m.			
8:00 a.m. to noon			
Noon to 4:00 p.m.			
4:00 to 8:00 p.m.			
8:00 p.m. to midnight			
		Total minutes of activity:	Total minutes of inactivity:

Reprinted from S. Blair, A. Dunn, B. Marcus, R.A. Carpenter, and P. Jaret, 2001, *Active Living Every Day* (Champaign, IL: Human Kinetics), 184.

My Personal Contract

For the week of _____, I, (your name) _____
_____, will do the following tasks to increase my physical activity.

Day	What I will do
Sunday	
Monday	
Tuesday	
Wednesday	
Thursday	
Friday	
Saturday	

When I complete the activities listed above, I will reward myself as follows:

_____

_____

I will involve _____ in my plan as follows: _____

_____

_____

_____

_____

_____

_____

Signed:_____ Date:_____

Witness:_____ Date:_____

References

Introduction

1. Prochaska, J.O., and DiClemente, C.C. 1983. Stages and processes of self-change of smoking: Toward an integrative model of change. *Journal of Consulting and Clinical Pyschology,* 51:390-395.

2. Prochaska, J.O., and B.H. Marcus. 1994. The transtheoretical model: Application to exercise. In *Exercise adherence: Its impact on public health,* ed. R.K. Dishman. Champaign, IL: Human Kinetics.

3. Marcus B.H., and L.H. Forsyth. 2003. *Motivating people to be physically active.* Champaign, IL: Human Kinetics.

Chapter 1

1. Blair, S., A.L. Dunn, B.H. Marcus, R.A. Carpenter, P. Jaret. 2001. *Active living every day.* Champaign, IL: Human Kinetics.

2. Centers for Disease Control and Prevention. 2004. Prevalence of no leisure-time physical activity—35 states and the District of Columbia, 1988-2002. *Morbidity and Mortality Weekly Report* 53(4):82-86 (Feb. 6).

3. Beil, L. 1999. What is proper weight? Shake it up or go figure. *Dallas Morning News,* August 30.

4. American Association of Retired Persons (AARP). 2002. *Exercise attitudes and behaviors: A survey of adults 50-79.* Washington, DC, May.

5. Blair, S.N., J.B. Kampert, H.W. Kohl III, C.E. Barlow, C.A. Macera, R.S. Paffenbarger Jr., and L.W. Gibbons. 1996. Influences of cardiorespiratory fitness and other precursors on cardiovascular disease and all-cause mortality in men and women. *Journal of the American Medical Association* 276:205-210.

6. Lindsay, J., D. Laurin, R. Verreault, R. Hebert, B. Helliwell, G.B. Hill, and I. McDowell. 2002. Risk factors for Alzheimer's disease: A prospective analysis from the Canadian Study of Health and Aging. *American Journal of Epidemiology* 156:445-453.

7. Lee, C.D., Blair, S.N., and Jackson, A.S. 1999. Cardiorespiratory fitness, body composition, and all-cause and cardiovascular disease mortality in men. *American Journal of Clinical Nutrition* 69:373-380.

8. Franklin, B.A., J.M. Conviser, B. Stewart, J. Lasch, and G.C. Timmis. 2005. Sporadic exercise: A trigger for acute cardiovascular events? *Circulation* 102:II-612.

9. Franklin, B.A., K. Bonzheim, S. Gordon, et al. 1998. Safety of medically supervised outpatient cardiac rehabilitation exercise therapy: A 16-year follow-up. *Chest* 114:902-906.

10. Canada Society for Exercise Physiology. 2002. *Physical Activity Readiness Questionnaire (PAR-Q).*

Chapter 2

1. Ellis, A. 1973. *Humanistic psychotherapy: The rational-emotive approach.* New York: Julian Press.

2. Ellis, A. 1974. *Disputing irrational beliefs.* New York: Institute for Rational Living.

3. American Association of Retired Persons (AARP). 2002. *Exercise attitudes and behaviors: A survey of adults 50-79.* Washington, DC, May.

Chapter 3

1. Olshansky, S.J., L. Hayflick, and B.A. Carnes. 2002. No truth to the fountain of youth. *Scientific American,* June, 92-95.

2. Blair, S., A.L. Dunn, B.H. Marcus, R.A. Carpenter, P. Jaret. 2001. *Active living every day.* Champaign, IL: Human Kinetics.

Chapter 4

1. Paffenbarger, R.S., Jr., and I.M. Lee. 1998. A natural history of athleticism, health, and longevity. *Journal of Sports Science* 16:S31-S45.

2. Boreham, C.A., W.F. Wallace, and A. Nevill. 2000. Training effects of accumulated daily stair-climbing exercise in previously sedentary young women. *Preventive Medicine* 30(4):277-281.

Chapter 7

1. American Association of Retired Persons (AARP). 2002. *Exercise attitudes and behaviors: A survey of adults 50-79.* Washington, DC, May.

Chapter 9

1. Borg, G.V. 1998. Borg's perceived exertion and pain scales. Champaign, IL: Human Kinetics.

Chapter 10

National Institutes of Health, National Institute on Aging. n.d. *Exercise: A guide from the National Institute on Aging.* Publication No. NIH 99-4258.

Chapter 11

1. Marcus, B.H., et al. 2000. Physical activity behavior change: Issues in adoption and maintenance. *Health Psychology* 19(1) (Suppl.):32-41

2. McAuley, E. 1992. The role of efficacy cognition in the prediction of exercise behavior in middle-aged adults. *Journal of Behavioral Medicine* 77:115-122.

3. Dubbert, P.M., and B.A. Stetson. 1995. Exercise and physical activity. In *Handbook of health and rehabilitation psychology,* ed. A.J. Goreczny, 255-274. New York: Plenum.

Chapter 12

1. U.S. Bureau of the Census. 2004. International data base, table 10. Life expectancy at birth by sex.

2. U.S. Department of Health and Human Services, Public Health Service, Centers for Disease Control and Prevention, National Center for Chronic Disease Prevention and Health Promotion, Division of Nutrition and Physical Activity. 1999. *Promoting physical activity: A Guide for community action.* Champaign, IL: Human Kinetics.

Word Search Solutions

CHAPTER 1

```
C K Y J Z S G F J A A P I N R
W O S S E N I D A E R Q N O I
P N N F S S M J E E N N O T S
F Y P T N R N H P L K F I C K
S U U D E Y S A O G N X T U S
M T K O H M R T Y D D O E F O
H Z I M U A P E A Y D Z H D P
W O H F T C G L H G Z H E N A
S C X I E N Y G A E E Y N C Y
E F O V A N Q J B T D F E J
M N B H T C E T A W I C N G
V Z C F T Y R B L M O O E P U
H W P B T B V G Y L W V N N A
G K Q H F T F C O S P C W U N
G B A C T I O N R X K Y D J O
```

CHAPTER 2

```
S E K D P P B A M L C J P H E
T O X R I J I M P R J E T A Y
H M O C Q C R C G Z R Y B H E
G S L H U P L A Q F N X B I P
U Y Z J O A C E C N N V H S T H
O Z J O A C E C N N V H P S D
H L K S G N T S U I O C A W G
T H Z Z J I O Z T V S M Y O A
L E U G O L A I D R E N N I Q
S Y Q N N C S B T V J K Y X
M Y I N T O O A N A L Y Z E E
U S M W P T V E K K R D W D E
M B M F L C C O F U E S O L J
Z N Q G R Y S N O C D M R X K
I J E S G Q Z Z P D Z V B A N
```

CHAPTER 3

```
S T G E L R H L X X E I W L S
A N L A V P O J M Q M H O I I
F E O H G D S U F Q I S T P G
F V P I S I C Z Y T I B B Q
I E V M T C N Z L E R V H C P
R P A U L C Q G O H G S J L O
M P R A X V A P T O Q N O O Z
A K C J M U O R D E L A Y U F
T W T Q N R A O Z C Y L N J S
I J B L O O D P R E S S U R E
O G A S E L M H E S T E G I U
N X I T S T H G U O H T W L S
S S S Z I O Q E F Q R N C M R
E O L F U L O O S B X G S Z M
R Y Z U D W O E X X Q P V W V
```

CHAPTER 4

```
W T P N H J M U Y H G C I L B
C L I M B I N G S T A I R S S
G S Z M G A K N Y J S E Y T
U S T W E Y L Y D E X S Z U O
J J I N Y M F A I Y T H H O B
X Z N K E D A T N E R K C B T
M B M L S M I N P C T Q O T R
Z G F T P R T C A X E Z L R O
S H A A O M O I V G Y Y R H
M P L I B U Y Q M B E J A S
R N R N N A L E Z M T M J S
G P G T N K Q B L V O V E F G
D D E L E G A T E U D C B N K
O R Y A W A R A F K R A P D T
H L O H R Z C C E E X B L B K
```

CHAPTER 5

```
U A E M Y J C I Z T P D E V V
G N I T T I F L L E W T K P V
U E O T P D I E V X X G O Q B
W Z H I B M Z W B U D J R B H
J X Z A T I S L A O G L T E
C S G E N A T H M D J G S G A
N D J A L A R U E F Z S E A U
L W G O I U N D L T B A E V K
J R O S A E B K Y A M G E U
O S B D E M N E L H Y U H E U
E D K N M U F W J V E E V I J
Y L Y J I J C I C W P D R A A
J T T K X L R E W A R D S S J
W R P M Y I K D X X I Q B U E
Y X G W X B R A F X C D Z R N
```

CHAPTER 6

```
Y P P N V Y X A Q Y R Y V O J
L T N F L H W O K S E W A Y M
G N I L C Y C U Z B T I U I D
Z O K L H V F A Y M A O Z B Q
E P S W I M M I N G W C E B M
C A S E O B I Q H U W N B M M
V U E D L S I T Q A Y A R X V
H C L R Q C G X L B R U D I C
M I Z Y O N S K E Y G U N N K
F K J I E B I U N L L E N H T
S E R R C N I S M E F N C T
D S T A G I C Y H F E E Z B
B S S L G Z S Q K K T L H F K
X Y G N W H V G M C T Z I Z Z
L L C O O A H O V U O L P G R
```

231

CHAPTER 7

```
Y T E F A S H J I N E O O N T
S D D W P Y M F E C N U S O Q
R E Q U I P M E N T X T O I B
E E K L M X R E G H M D U A G
Z M T H Y B I G B F U O D C K
G Q O N A N B S Y E A O D C C
D W R H E W R E G V Q R P I T
T X C V X C Q N L O N S V F B
V H N C U L S P D L C J N I K
I O W J Y T S S Z Y S N N T K
C V X M A U U P E X W D R R Y
R E N I A R T L A N O S R E P
Z J G C A A H J J O T W J C P
T T V C N S G Y R Y A I U F X
D X X T Y P U S N O K R F E Y
```

CHAPTER 8

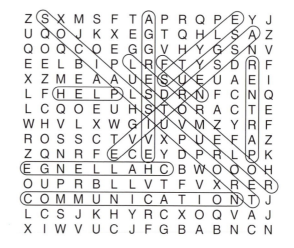

```
Z S X M S F T A P R Q P E Y J
U Q O J K X E G T Q H L S A Z
Q O Q C O E G G V H Y G S N V
E E L B I P L R F T Y S D R F
X Z M E A A U E S U E U A E I
L F H E L P L S D R N F C N Q
L C Q O E U H S T O R A C T E
W H V L X W G I U V M Z Y R A
R O S S C T V V X P U E F R P
Z Q N R F E C E Y D P R L P H
E G N E L L A H C B W O O O H
O U P R B L L V T F V X R E R
C O M M U N I C A T I O N T J
L C S J K H Y R C X O Q V A J
X I W V U C J F G B A B N C N
```

CHAPTER 9

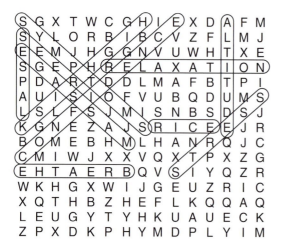

```
Y R G F L T X Q C A V H I T F
Z J V W A R M U P M Q G C R U
C J H F M A N G H K T A E T Z
G I Q L S I W P I Y R Q A G U
Y Y K O A N T B P T U Y E F X
R I H Q Z I N E N E P J Q L C
N J R M W N S O N T A U M T T
W O E M J G C C I X W K L C I
O R V X M Z Y Y C T B K M S M
D Q Z A N O F P Q P R L V C E
L T L T G N E D D J Q O E J E P
O N B R P E J M D O S S X U I
O L V W W O R C E Y B V S E K
C N H J U O P F C K C W U P V
Y T I S N E T N I W N I E M Z
```

CHAPTER 10

```
D R I U L A T J N R Q K A R S
Y O P W E R E V E Q V X S U E
J T G Q A C P S G F W Q T B T
G O R U N V T K X V B X B B S
D L J A A S I K Y L C G G E A
Y L L H T X D O S X X W J R L
M A E A T H G I E W Y D O B N
B M N H E K Z A N S H E P A O
O C V R D K Z Z I U P H L N Q
E X E P P N C A H C B E O R K
S P U F W K A W C B S E R S W
S T R E T C H H A E E I Y T T
F F Q U D V W Z M Y G G E R S
M O N Z O N L D V W I B P M A
R W B Z V P U G U U L F R E L
```

CHAPTER 11

```
S G X T W C G H I E X D A F M
S Y L O R B I B C V Z F L M J
E E M J H G G N V U W H T X E
S G E P H R E L A X A T I O N
P D A R T D L M A F B T P I
A U I S I O F V U B Q D U M S
L S L F S J M S N B S D S J
K G N E Z A J S R I C E E J R
B O M E B H M L H A N R Q J C
C M I W J X X V Q X T P X Z G
E H T A E R B Q V S I Y Q Z R
W K H G X W I J G E U Z R I C
X Q T H B Z H E F L K Q Q A Q
L E U G Y T Y H K U A U E C K
Z P X D K P H Y M D P L Y I M
```

Index

Note: The italicized *f* and *t* following page numbers refers to figures and tables, respectively.

A

aches and pains 14-15
action-oriented approach xviii
action stage xiii*t*, xvi*f*, 3*t*, 208
activities of daily living 9, 10
advocates for physical activity 220-224
aerobic fitness
    balanced fitness and 188-191
    chapter checklist on 111
    defined 90-91, 97
    stationary cycling 106-108, 189*t*
    summary on 111
    walking 98-102, 189*t*
    water activities 102-106, 189*t*
aerobic fitness program
    chapter checklist on 153-154
    description of 147-149
    FITT plan and 140-145, 147
    goals for 149-150*f*
    personal contract for 151*f*-152*f*
    summary on 153
    walking test 152-153*f*
affirmations 48-49*f*, 82, 87
aging
    blood pressure and 38-40, 45*t*
    causes of 37
    muscle loss and 38, 40
    osteoarthritis and 42-44, 47*t*
    osteoporosis and 41-42, 47*t*
    signs of 36*f*
altitude sickness 202-203
Alzheimer's disease 11
angina 13*t*, 45*t*
approval 27
arched back stretch 184
arm raise 171
arthritis
    aging and 37, 180
    heat and cold for 178
    myth buster 11
    osteoarthritis 9-10, 42-44, 47*t*
    precautions and tips 47*t*
assertive communication 133-136
asthma 46*t*
atherosclerosis 39, 45*t*
athlete's foot 74*t*

B

back pain 47*t*
back stretch 184
balance
    defined 93
    exercises to improve 162, 189*t*
    tests 93*f*-94*f*, 163*f*
balance and time management 61-63
balanced fitness program 188-191
benefits of physical activity
    bone strength 7*t*, 9
    cancer risk reduction 7*t*, 9, 91
    diabetes risk reduction 7*t*, 8, 91
    list of 6, 7*t*
    longevity 7*t*-8*f*
    restful sleep 7*t*, 10
    weight control 7*t*, 10, 11-12, 40
    well-being 7*t*, 10-11
biceps curl
    with handheld weights 175
    with resistance rubber bands 176
blood pressure 38-40, 45*t*
body composition 40, 94-95
body fat 12*f*, 40
body weight activities 157, 160, 165, 189*t*
bone and joint problems 41-44, 47*t*
bone density testing 42
bone strength
    osteoporosis and 41-42
    physical activity and 7*t*, 9
bones, broken 7*t*, 15, 41, 42
Borg scale of perceived exertion 144*t*, 154, 158
breathing, deep 210-211
bunions 74*t*

C

calcium 41-42, 47*t*
calendar reminders 78
calf raise 170
calf stretch 181-182
calories burned during daily tasks 5*t*-6*t*
cancer 7*t*, 9, 37, 48*t*, 91
cardiovascular disease
    death rates from 8*f*
    heart attacks 7*t*, 13-14, 45*t*, 198
    precautions and tips 45*t*, 46*t*
chair stand 166
change
    path toward xv-xvi*f*
    Readiness to Change Questionnaire 2*f*-3*f*, 109-110*t*, 206, 207
    skills for xiv, xv*t*, 218*f*
    stages of xii-xiv, xviii*t*, 207-208
changes, major life 216-220*f*
chest fly 172-173
chest press with resistance rubber band 173
chronic obstructive pulmonary disease (COPD) 46*t*
clothing 76, 79, 80
commitments
    family responsibilities 199
    reviewing 60-61
    social activities 200
    work 200-201
communication, assertive 133-136
community action 220-224
community resources 120-121
confidence level 110*t*, 194-195*f*
congestive heart failure 46*t*
contemplation stage xiii*t*, xvi*f*, 2, 3*t*, 207
contract, personal
    for aerobic exercise 151*f*-152*f*
    for increasing physical activity 84*f*-85*f*, 228*f*
cool-down and warm-up 145-147, 189

corns and calluses 73, 74*t*
coronary heart disease 45*t*. *See also* heart attacks
cues and prompts 78-80*f*, 110*t*
cycling, stationary 106-108, 189*t*

D

daily tasks
 activities of daily living 9, 10
 calories burned during 5*t*-6*t*
death
 delaying 7-8*f*
 sudden 13-14
dehydration 76-78
depression 7*t*, 11, 180
diabetes
 aging and 37
 foot care and 74-75
 precautions and tips 17, 48*t*
 risk reduction 7*t*, 8, 11, 91
 weight and 40
doctor, questions for 17-18

E

equipment
 handheld weights 117-118, 160-161, 165
 large 118-120*f*
 resistance rubber bands, 118, 160-161, 165
 small 116-118
 swimming 104
 weight machines 161
excuses 29*f*-30*f*
exercise, aerobic
 chapter checklist on 111
 defined 90-91, 97
 stationary cycling 106-108, 189*t*
 summary on 111
 walking 98-102, 189*t*
 water activities 102-106, 189*t*
exercise dropouts 208
exercises, strength building
 balance and 162-163*f*
 body weight activities 157, 160, 165
 leg and hip exercises 165*f*-170
 types of 158-163
 upper body exercises 170-177
exertion, perceived 144*t*, 158

F

failure xvii, 24-25
family responsibilities 199
fitness balls 118
fitness centers 122-124
fitness equipment
 description of 116-120*f*
 handheld weights 117-118, 160-161, 165
 resistance rubber bands 118, 160-161, 165
 weight machines 161
fitness products 126-127
FITT plan
 aerobic fitness and 147-153*f*
 defined 140
 frequency (F) 141, 158*t*
 intensity (I) 141*t*-145, 158*t*
 muscle fitness and 157-158*t*
 time (T) 145, 158*t*
flexibility
 checking 92*f*-93*f*
 defined 43, 157, 178
flexibility exercises. *See also* stretching
 in balanced fitness program 188-191
 guidelines for 178-180

importance of 43, 178
 for major muscle groups and joints 181-185
foot care 73-75
forward reach test 94*f*
fractures 7*t*, 9, 15, 41, 42, 47*t*
fun and humor 136-137

G

goal setting
 for aerobic exercise 149-150*f*
 personal contracts 84*f*-85*f*, 151*f*-152*f*, 228*f*
 short-term goals 83, 217
 tips 84

H

habits, reshaping xi-xviii
hamstring stretch 181
handheld weights and resistance rubber bands
 description of 117-118, 160-161
 tips on using 165
health benefits of physical activity
 bone strength 7*t*, 9
 cancer risk reduction 7*t*, 9
 diabetes risk reduction 7*t*, 8
 list of 6, 7*t*
 longevity 7*t*-8*f*
 restful sleep 7*t*, 10
 weight control 7*t*, 10, 11-12, 40
 well-being 7*t*, 10-11
health clubs 122-124
heart attacks 7*t*, 13-14, 45*t*, 198
heart disease 8*f*, 17, 37, 39, 45*t*, 46*t*, 91
heart rate, maximum 143
heart rate monitors 117
heat stroke 77, 78
high blood pressure 17, 39, 40, 45*t*, 91
hip extension 167-168
hip flexion 167
home, physical activity at
 advantages of 114-115
 equipment for 116-120
 questions about 116
 short bouts of 64
housework 5*t*, 10, 64, 90, 115

I

ice packs 178, 197
illness
 activity and 196-199
 special health problems 44-48*t*
inactive lifestyles 4-5
influencing others 219-220
injury
 RICE for treating 196, 197
 risk of 13, 14-15
 ways to stay active after 196
intensity of exercise 140*t*, 141*t*-145, 158*t*
irrational thinking
 changing your 25-27
 excuses 29*f*-30*f*
 irrational ideas 27*f*
 substituting rational ideas 28*f*

J

joint flexibility 43, 92*f*-93*f*, 157, 158*t*. *See also* stretching
joint pain 9-10, 41, 42-44, 47*t*

K

knee extension 168-169
knee flexion 169

L

lapses and relapses
  as common challenge 194
  dealing with xv*t*, xvi*f*
  getting back on track 206-208
  high-risk situations 203*f*-206
  prevention of 209*f*
leg and back stretch 183
leg and hip exercises 165*f*-170
leg strength test 165*f*-166*f*
life expectancy 220*t*
lifestyle physical activity
  building strength with 160
  defined xii
  structured aerobic fitness versus 140*t*
  ways to fit in 64-66*f*

M

maintenance stage xiii*t*, xiv, xvi*f*, 3*t*
massage 212
memory, improved 7*t*, 10-11
menopause 36*f*, 41, 42
model program
  for aerobic fitness 147-153*f*
  for balanced fitness 188-191
mood, improvement in 10-11
motivation
  affirmations 48-49*f*, 82, 87
  persistence and xvii
  rewards 81*f*-83*f*, 110*t*
muscle endurance 91, 157
muscle fitness
  defined 91
  leg and hip exercises for 165*f*-170
  strength building terminology 157
  upper body exercises for 170-177
muscle strength 91, 92*f*, 157

N

neck roll 212
neck stretch 185

O

obesity
  precautions and tips 48*t*
  risk of death and 12*f*
  weight control 7*t*, 11-12, 40
organizing for an active lifestyle
  chapter checklist on 86-87
  clothing 76, 79, 80, 163
  cues and prompts 78-80*f*
  dehydration prevention 76-78
  foot care 73-75
  rewards 81*f*-83*f*, 110*t*
  shoes 48*t*, 70-73
  short-term goals 83-84, 217
  summary on 86
orthotics 74
osteoarthritis
  description of 42-44
  heat and cold for 178
  myth buster 11
  physical activity and 9-10, 43
  precautions and tips 47*t*
osteoporosis 41-42*f*, 47*t*
overheating 76-78

P

past successes 22-24*f*
pedometers 54-56*f*, 117

perfectionism 27
peripheral vascular disease 45*t*
persistence
  getting back on track 206-208
  motivation and xvii
  prevention of lapses 209*f*
personal contracts
  for aerobic exercise 151*f*-152*f*
  for increasing physical activity 84*f*-85*f*, 228*f*
personal time study 57*f*-60, 227*f*
personal trainers 125-126*f*
physical activity
  advocates for 220-224
  balanced fitness program 188-191
  benefits of 6-12
  decline in 4-6*t*
  exercise versus 90
  pros and cons of 30-32*f*, 86, 225*f*
  questions for doctor about 17-18
  risks of 13-15
  small steps 32-33
  thoughts about 18-19, 50*f*-51*f*, 226*f*
Physical Activity Readiness Questionnaire (PAR-Q) 15, 16*f*, 17
places to be active
  community resources 120-121, 220-224
  fitness centers 122-124
  home 114-120*f*
precontemplation stage xiii*t*, xvi*f*, 2, 3*t*, 207
preparation stage xiii*t*, xvi*f*, 2, 207-208
progressive muscle relaxation 211
pros and cons of physical activity 30-32*f*, 86, 225*f*
pulse rate 142*f*-143*f*

Q

questionnaires
  Physical Activity Readiness Questionnaire (PAR-Q) 15, 16*f*, 17
  Readiness to Change Questionnaire 2*f*-3*f*, 109-110*t*, 206, 207
questions for doctor 17-18
questions for personal trainers 126*f*
quick-fix programs xi, xviii*t*

R

rainwear 76
Readiness to Change Questionnaire 2*f*-3*f*, 109-110*t*, 206, 207
relaxation techniques 210-213*f*
reminders 78-80*f*
resistance rubber bands
  description of 118, 160-161
  tips on using 165
rewards 81*f*-83*f*, 110*t*
RICE method 196, 197

S

seated row with resistance rubber band 174
self-paced program xiv-xvi
sex, better 7
shoes 48*t*, 70-73
short bouts of activity 64-66*f*
short-term goals 83-84, 217
shoulder flexion 171
shoulder shrugs 212
sickness
  activity and 196-199
  special health problems 44-48*t*
side leg raise 169-170
side shoulder raise 172
side steps 146-147

skill power xiv
skills for making changes xiv, xv*t*, 218*f*
sleep, restful 7*t*, 10
smoking 17, 23-24, 37, 42, 46*t*
social activities 200
sport, picking a 186-188*f*
sprains 15, 70, 196, 197
spurs 74*t*
stair climbing 54, 56
stationary cycling 106-108
step counters 54-56*f*, 117
strength building
    balance exercises and 162-163*f*
    in balanced fitness program 188-191
    body weight activities 157, 160, 165
    handheld weights for 117-118, 160-161, 165
    leg and hip exercises 165*f*-170
    resistance rubber bands for 118, 160-161, 165
    techniques and tips 163-164
    terminology 157
    types of exercises for 158-163
    upper body exercises 170-177
    weight machines for 161
stress fractures 15
stress management
    relaxation techniques 210-213*f*
    tips 210
stress reduction 7
stretching
    in balanced fitness program 188-191
    exercises for major muscle groups and joints 181-185
    getting up from the floor 179-181
    muscle fitness and 157-158*t*
    relaxation and 211-212
    techniques and tips 178-179
    terminology 157-158
strong bones
    osteoporosis and 41-42
    physical activity and 7*t*, 9
structured aerobic fitness 90, 140*t*, 189*t*
structured exercise xii, 90, 189*t*
success
    past successes 22-24*f*
    predictors of xvii
support system 130-133
swimming
    benefits of 102-103
    equipment 104
    safety tips 105-106

T

tai chi move 146
talk test 145
television 5*t*, 19, 79, 80, 95, 107, 201
tennis shoes 70-71
thinking and feeling skills 110*t*
thinking patterns
    changing your 25-27
    excuses 29*f*-30*f*
    irrational ideas 27*f*
    substituting rational ideas 28*f*
thoughts
    learning from 50*f*-51*f*, 226*f*
    recording 50*f*, 226*f*
time management
    balance 61-63
    chapter checklist on 67
    commitments 60-61, 199-201
    fitting in fitness 64-66*f*
    personal time study 57*f*-60, 227*f*
    priorities 56-57

    summary on 67, 110*t*
    tips 63-64
toenails 73, 74*t*
trainers, personal 125-126*f*
training zone 142*f*-143*f*
travel 65, 201-203
triceps extension
    with handheld weights 175-176
    with resistance rubber bands 177
triceps stretch 182
trunk stretch 185
type 1 diabetes 48*t*
type 2 diabetes
    foot care and 74-75
    precautions and tips 17, 48*t*
    risk reduction 7*t*, 8, 11, 91
    weight and 40

U

unsuccessful attempts 24-25
upper body exercises 170-177

V

vacations 65, 201-203
valvular heart disease 46*t*
videos 117
visualization 211
vitamin D 41, 42, 47*t*

W

walking
    balanced fitness and 189, 191
    calories burned while 5*t*, 6*t*
    events 188
    at home 64, 79, 115
    reasons to walk 98
    safety tips 101-102
    step counters 54-56*f*
    techniques and tips 99-100
    two-minute walk 33
    types of 99
    on vacations 65, 203-204
    variations of 100-101
    at work 64-65
walking shoes 70, 80, 201
walking test 152-153*f*
warm-up and cool-down 145-147, 189
water 48*t*, 77, 78, 79, 101, 106, 108
water activities
    swimming 102-104
    techniques and tips for 105-106
    water aerobics 104-105
weighing pros and cons 30-32*f*, 86, 225*f*
weight control 7*t*, 11-12, 40
weight machines 161
willpower xiv
women
    heart attacks in 198
    life expectancy of 220*t*
    menopause 36*f*, 41, 42
word searches 20, 34, 52, 87, 112, 128, 138, 154, 192, 214
word search solutions 231-232
work commitments 200-201
wrist stretch 183

Y

youth, remembering your 95-97

About the Authors

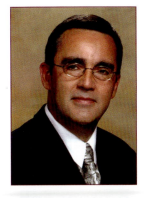

Walter Ettinger, MD, is a physician and university professor with a specialty in gerontology. He is also president of the University of Massachusetts Memorial Medical Center. A board-certified specialist in aging and the muscle and bone systems, Ettinger is a nationally recognized researcher, teacher, and clinician in these areas. He also published the seminal article demonstrating the importance and safety of exercise in people with arthritis.

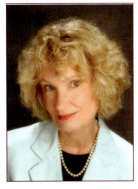

Brenda Wright, PhD, is the vice president for program development for INTERVENT USA and a health promotion consultant. For 12 years she served as director of behavioral science and health promotion at The Cooper Institute in Dallas. There, she developed comprehensive lifestyle management programs for delivery at worksites, health and fitness centers, clinics and hospitals, and government agencies. She has also developed patient education materials for the Baylor Senior Health Centers in Dallas as well as health promotion programs for assisted living centers in Washington, Florida, and Texas. In 2002, Wright received the Distinguished Alumni Award in human ecology from the University of Texas at Austin.

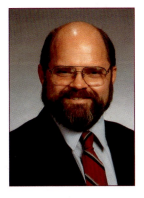

Steven Blair, PED, is president and CEO of The Cooper Institute and is one of the world's most eminent epidemiologists in the area of physical activity and health. He is the lead author of many of the landmark research studies about the benefits of exercise. Blair was senior scientific editor of the U.S. Surgeon General's Report on Physical Activity and Health, and he received the Surgeon General's Medallion for his work. He has also served as the president of the American College of Sports Medicine (ACSM) and the National Coalition for Promoting Physical Activity. Blair has three honorary doctorates, a 1994 doctor honoris causa from the Free University of Brussels, a 1996 doctor of health science from Lander University, and a 2002 doctor of health science honoris causa from the University of Bristol (UK).

All three authors are over 50 years of age.

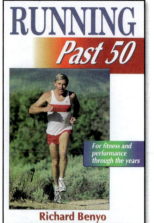
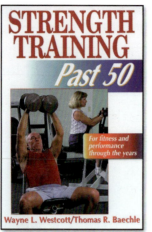
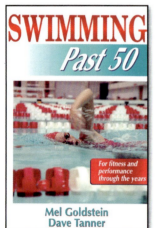
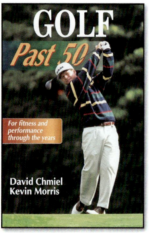
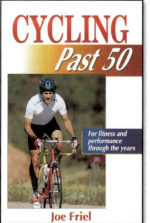
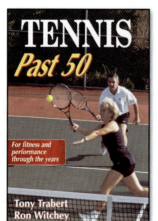
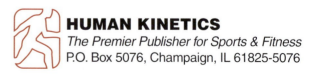